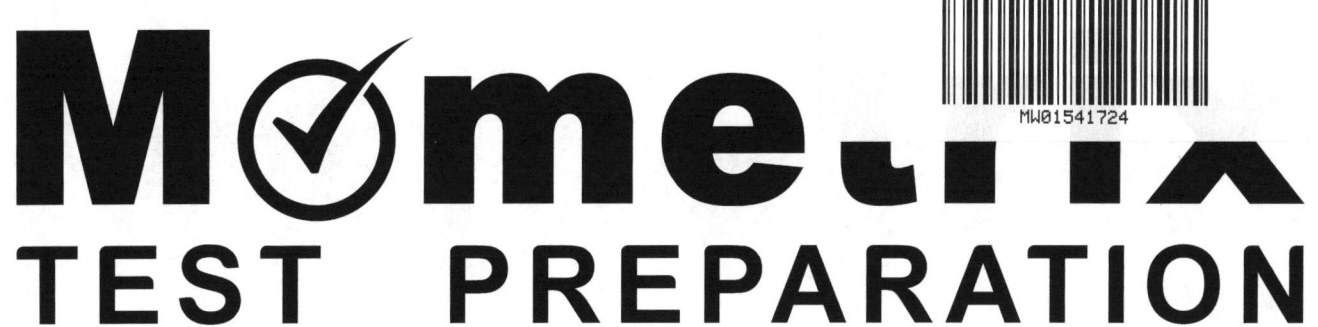

Adult-Gerontology Primary Care Nurse Practitioner Exam
Secrets Study Guide
Part 2 of 2

Dear Future Exam Success Story

First of all, **THANK YOU** for purchasing Mometrix study materials!

Second, congratulations! You are one of the few determined test-takers who are committed to doing whatever it takes to excel on your exam. **You have come to the right place.** We developed these study materials with one goal in mind: to deliver you the information you need in a format that's concise and easy to use.

In addition to optimizing your guide for the content of the test, we've outlined our recommended steps for breaking down the preparation process into small, attainable goals so you can make sure you stay on track.

We've also analyzed the entire test-taking process, identifying the most common pitfalls and showing how you can overcome them and be ready for any curveball the test throws you.

Standardized testing is one of the biggest obstacles on your road to success, which only increases the importance of doing well in the high-pressure, high-stakes environment of test day. Your results on this test could have a significant impact on your future, and this guide provides the information and practical advice to help you achieve your full potential on test day.

Your success is our success

We would love to hear from you! If you would like to share the story of your exam success or if you have any questions or comments in regard to our products, please contact us at **800-673-8175** or **support@mometrix.com**.

Thanks again for your business and we wish you continued success!

Sincerely,
The Mometrix Test Preparation Team

Need more help? Check out our flashcards at:
http://mometrixflashcards.com/NP

Copyright © 2022 by Mometrix Media LLC. All rights reserved.
Written and edited by the Mometrix Exam Secrets Test Prep Team
Printed in the United States of America

Table of Contents

Plan of Care: Implementation and Evaluation (continued) — 1
- Gastrointestinal Procedures and Interventions — 1
- Genitourinary Pathophysiology — 4
- Genitourinary Procedures and Interventions — 11
- Bowel and Bladder Training — 14
- Neurological Pathophysiology — 16
- Respiratory Pathophysiology — 26
- Respiratory Procedures and Interventions — 38
- Hematologic Pathophysiology — 43
- Hematologic Procedures and Interventions — 48
- Immunologic and Oncologic Pathophysiology — 50
- Integumentary Pathophysiology — 58
- Integumentary Procedures and Interventions — 61
- Musculoskeletal Pathophysiology — 62
- Multisystem Pathophysiology — 66
- Acid Base Imbalances — 76
- Electrolyte Imbalances — 79
- Infection Control — 82
- Infectious Diseases — 84
- Psychosocial Pathophysiology — 92
- Psychosocial Procedures and Interventions — 100
- Geriatric Pathophysiology — 100
- Alternative, Complementary, and Non-Pharmacologic Interventions — 106
- Care Coordination and Collaboration — 113
- Telehealth — 120
- Education Theory — 123
- Principles of Education — 124

Professional Practice — 133
- Scope and Standards of Practice of the Advanced Practice Nurse — 133
- APRN Billing, Reimbursement, and Insurance — 135
- Ethics — 136
- Patient Rights — 139
- Legal Regulations — 140
- Abuse and Neglect — 143
- Health Promotion and Disease Prevention — 149

NP Primary Care Practice Test — 154

Answer Key and Explanations — 162

How to Overcome Test Anxiety — 170
- Causes of Test Anxiety — 170
- Elements of Test Anxiety — 171
- Effects of Test Anxiety — 171
- Physical Steps for Beating Test Anxiety — 172
- Mental Steps for Beating Test Anxiety — 173

STUDY STRATEGY	174
TEST TIPS	176
IMPORTANT QUALIFICATION	177

TELL US YOUR STORY **178**

ADDITIONAL BONUS MATERIAL **179**

Plan of Care: Implementation and Evaluation (continued)

Gastrointestinal Procedures and Interventions

NG TUBES, SUMP TUBES, AND LEVIN TUBES

Nasogastric **(NG) tubes** are plastic or vinyl tubes inserted through the nose, down the esophagus, and into the stomach. **Sump tubes** are radiopaque with a vent lumen to prevent a vacuum from forming with high suction. **Levin tubes** have no vent lumen and are used only with low suction. NG tubes drain gastric secretions, allow sampling of secretions, or provide access to the stomach and upper GI tract. They are used for lavage after medication overdose, for decompression, and for instillation of medications or fluids. NG tubes are contraindicated with obstruction proximal to the stomach or gastric pathology, such as hemorrhage.

Tube-insertion length is estimated: earlobe to xiphoid + earlobe to nose tip + 15 cm.

The tube is inserted through the naris with the patient upright, if possible, and swallowing sips of water. Vasoconstrictors and topical anesthetic reduce gag reflex. Placement is checked with insufflation of air or aspiration of stomach contents and verified by x-ray. The NG is secured and drainage bag provided. Tubes attached to continuous low or intermittent high suction must be monitored frequently.

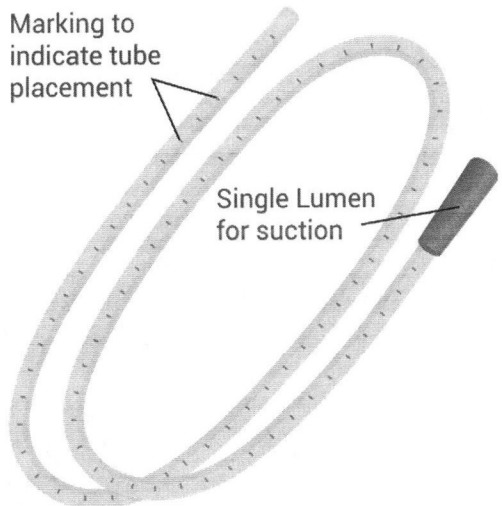

Levin Tube

PEG TUBE

Percutaneous endoscopic gastrostomy (PEG), used for tube feedings, involves intubation of the esophagus with the endoscope and insertion of a sheathed needle with a guidewire through the abdomen and stomach wall so that a catheter can be fed down the esophagus, snared, and pulled out through the opening where the needle was inserted and secured. The PEG tube should not be secured to the abdomen until the PEG is fully healed, which usually takes 2 to 4 weeks, because tension caused by taping the tube against the abdomen may cause the tract to change shape and direction. The tract should be straight to facilitate insertion and removal of catheters. Once the tract has healed, the original PEG tube can generally be replaced with a balloon gastrostomy tube. External stabilizing devices can be applied to the skin to hold the tube in place but should be placed 1 to 2 cm above the skin surface to prevent excessive tension that may result in buried bumper syndrome (BBS) in which the internal fixation device becomes lodged in the mucosal lining of the gastric wall, resulting in ulceration.

Drains

The following are different types of drains a patient may have, including pertinent nursing considerations:

- **Simple drains** are latex or vinyl tubes of varying sizes/lengths. They are usually placed through a stab wound near the area of involvement.
- **Penrose drains** are flat, soft rubber/latex tubes placed in surgical wounds to drain fluid by gravity and capillary action.

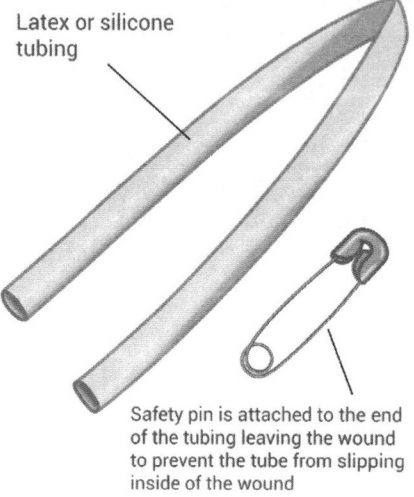

Latex or silicone tubing

Safety pin is attached to the end of the tubing leaving the wound to prevent the tube from slipping inside of the wound

- **Sump drains** are double-lumen or tri-lumen tubes (with a third lumen for infusions). The multiple lumens produce venting when air enters the inflow lumen and forces drainage out of the large lumen.
- **A percutaneous drainage catheter** is inserted into the wound to provide continuous drainage for infection/fluid collection. Irrigation of the catheter may be required to maintain patency. Skin barriers and pouching systems may also be necessary.

SAFE PERCUTANEOUS DRAINAGE KIT

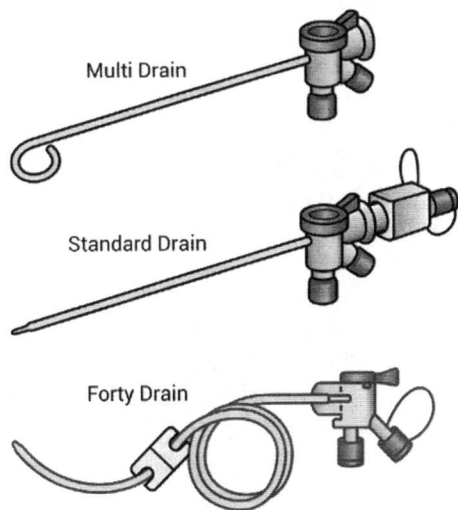

- **Closed drainage systems** use low-pressure suction to provide continuous gravity drainage of wounds. Drains are attached to collapsible suction reservoirs that provide negative pressure. The nurse must remember to always re-establish negative pressure after emptying these drains. There are two types in frequent use:
  - *Jackson-Pratt® is* a bulb-type drain that is about the size of a lemon. A thin plastic drain from the wound extends to a squeeze bulb that can hold about 100 mL of drainage.

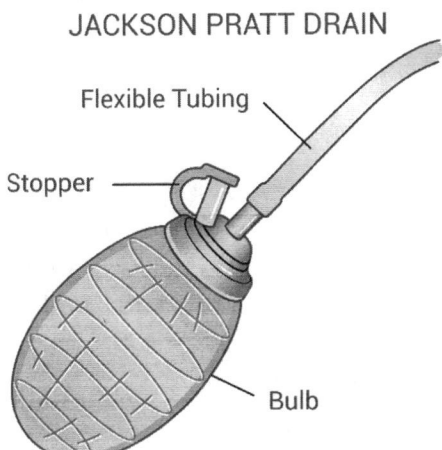

  - *Hemovac®* is a round drain with coiled springs inside that are compressed after emptying to create suction. The device can hold up to 500 mL of drainage.

DETERMINING THE CALORIC REQUIREMENTS OF CRITICALLY ILL PATIENTS

When an individual requires hospitalization for a critical illness, his or her **caloric requirements** must be determined so that normal body function is maintained, and so that recovery is as quick as possible. There are many factors that must be considered when attempting to determine the requirements of an ill patient. First, the **age** of the patient is important. If the patient is a growing child or adolescent, he or she will have very different nutritional requirements than an elderly individual would have. Also, to be considered is the **physical and nutritional status** of the patient, independent of the illness. A patient who is normally very active would have different requirements than an overweight, sedentary individual. Along the same lines, **comorbidities**, such as diabetes and atherosclerosis, need to be considered, as well as overall **stress levels** of the patient.

ENTERAL SUPPORT AND PARENTERAL SUPPORT

Enteral nutrition is a method of providing nutrition to a patient through a tube; the tube may be placed in either the nose (a nasogastric tube), the stomach (a percutaneous endoscopic gastrostomy [PEG] tube), or the small bowel (a percutaneous endoscopic jejunal [J] tube). When the tube has been placed, nutrition can be administered through the tube and absorbed by the patient's digestive system. Various **enteric formulas** exist, and the choice is dependent on the nutritional requirements of the patient.

Parenteral nutrition (also called total parenteral nutrition [**TPN**]) is a method of providing nutrition that completely bypasses the digestive system by administering nutrition through an intravenous line. Enteral support is the preferred method of providing nutrition, although in patients suffering from some compromise of the gastrointestinal tract, parenteral nutrition is the only option.

TROUBLE-SHOOTING PROBLEMS RELATED TO ENTERAL FEEDINGS

Feeding tubes are commonly found in the critical care setting, as many patients are intubated and unable to take oral nutrition or medication. General maintenance involves checking placement before flushing anything into the tube (prevents aspiration), flushing the tubes with at least 30 mL of water before and after use, and every 4 hours. Never crush enteric-coated medications, and keep the HOB inclined at least 30° at all times during feeding. **Complications** include:

- **Vomiting/aspiration:** Caused by incorrect placement, gastric emptying, and/or formula intolerance.
    - o Treatment: Confirm placement by checking pH (preferred to air bolus); delay feeding one hour and check residual volume before resuming. Refrigerate formula, check expiration, and use only for 24 hours.
- **Diarrhea:** Caused by rapid feeding, antibiotics/medications, intolerance of formula or hypertonic formula, and/or tube migration.
    - o Treatment: Reduce rate of feeding, evaluate medications, avoid hanging feedings longer than 8 hours, and add fiber or decrease sodium in the feed.
- **Displacement of tube:**
    - o Treatment: For NG tube, replace using the other nostril, only if not surgically placed. For G-tube or J-tube, cover the site and notify the physician.
    - o Prevention: secure all tubes with the appropriate device and mark placement to identify migration.
- **Tube occlusion:**
    - o Treatment: Check for kinks and obvious problems. Aspirate fluid, instill warm water, and aspirate to loosen occlusion. The physician may order an enzyme or sodium bicarb solution.

Genitourinary Pathophysiology

INCONTINENCE

Urinary incontinence occurs more commonly in women than men and can range from an intermittent leaking of urine to a full loss of bladder control. Causes of urinary incontinence may include neurologic injury (including cerebral vascular accidents), infections, weakness of the muscles of the bladder and certain medications including diuretics, antihistamines, and antidepressants. **Stress incontinence** is defined as an involuntary leakage of urine with sneezing, coughing, laughing, lifting, or exercising. **Urge incontinence** is defined as an uncontrollable need to urinate on a frequent basis. **Total incontinence** is the full loss of bladder control.

Signs and symptoms: Urinary frequency and urgency may accompany the inability to control urine. If urinary incontinence is severe, incontinence associated dermatitis may occur, predisposing the patient to skin breakdown and the development of pressure ulcers.

Diagnosis: Physical assessment and presence of symptoms. Ultrasound, urinalysis, urodynamic testing, and cystoscopy may be used to determine the underlying cause.

Treatment: Treatment options are dependent on the type of urinary incontinence and the severity. Bladder training and pelvic muscle exercises may be utilized to strengthen muscles to control leakage of urine. In female patients with stress incontinence, a vaginal pessary may be inserted into the vagina to help support the bladder. Suburethral slings may also be surgically implanted to support the urethra. Anticholinergics, antispasmodics, and tricyclic antidepressants may also be used in the treatment of urinary incontinence.

HYDRONEPHROSIS

Hydronephrosis is a symptom of a disease involving swelling of the kidney pelvises and calyces because of an obstruction that causes urine to be retained in the kidney. In chronic conditions, symptoms may be delayed until severe kidney damage has occurred. Over time, the kidney begins to atrophy. The primary conditions that predispose to hydronephrosis include:

- Vesicoureteral reflux
- Obstruction at the ureteropelvic junction
- Renal edema (non-obstructive)
- Any condition that impairs drainage of the ureters can cause backup of the urine

Symptoms vary widely depending upon cause and whether the condition is acute or chronic.

- Acute episodes are usually characterized by flank pain, abnormal creatinine and electrolyte levels, and increased pH.
- The enlarged kidney may be palpable as a soft mass.

Treatment includes:

- Identifying the cause of obstruction and correcting it to ensure adequate drainage.
- A nephrostomy tube, ureteral stent or pyeloplasty may be done surgically in some cases.
- A urinary catheter may be inserted if there is outflow obstruction from the bladder.

RENAL AND URETERAL CALCULI

Renal and urinary calculi occur frequently, more commonly in males, and can relate to diseases (hyperparathyroidism, renal tubular acidosis, gout) and lifestyle factors, such as sedentary work. Calculi can form at any age, most composed of calcium, and can range in size from very tiny to larger than 6 mm. Those smaller than 4 mm can usually pass in the urine easily.

Diagnostic studies include clinical findings, UA, pregnancy test to rule out ectopic pregnancy, BUN and creatinine if indicated, ultrasound (for pregnant women and children), IV urography. Helical CT (non-contrast) is diagnostic.

Symptoms occur with obstruction and are usually of sudden onset and acute:

- Severe flank pain radiating to abdomen and ipsilateral testicle or labium majus, abdominal or pelvic pain (young children)
- Nausea and vomiting
- Diaphoresis
- Hematuria

Treatment includes:

- Instructions and equipment for straining urine
- Antibiotics if concurrent infection
- Extracorporeal shock-wave lithotripsy
- Surgical removal: percutaneous/standard nephrolithotomy
- Analgesia: opiates and NSAIDs

ACUTE TUBULAR NECROSIS

Acute tubular necrosis (ATN) occurs when a hypoxic condition causes renal ischemia that damages tubular cells of the glomeruli so they are unable to adequately filter the urine, leading to acute renal failure. Causes include hypotension, hyperbilirubinemia, sepsis, surgery (especially cardiac or vascular), and birth complications. ATN may result from nephrotoxic injury related to obstruction or drugs, such as chemotherapy, acyclovir, and antibiotics, such as sulfonamides and streptomycin. Symptoms may be non-specific initially and can include life-threatening complications.

Symptoms include:

- Lethargy
- Nausea and vomiting
- Hypovolemia with low cardiac output and generalized vasodilation
- Fluid and electrolyte imbalance leading to hypertension, CNS abnormalities, metabolic acidosis, arrhythmias, edema, and congestive heart failure
- Uremia leading to destruction of platelets and bleeding, neurological deficits, and disseminated intravascular coagulopathy (DIC)
- Infections, including pericarditis and sepsis

Treatment includes:

- Identifying and treating underlying cause, discontinuing nephrotoxic agents
- Supportive care
- Loop diuretics (in some cases), such as Lasix®
- Antibiotics for infection (can include pericarditis and sepsis)
- Kidney dialysis

ACUTE KIDNEY INJURY

Acute kidney injury (AKI), previously known as acute renal failure, is an acute disruption of kidney function that results in decreased renal perfusion, a decrease in glomerular filtration rate and a buildup of metabolic waste products (azotemia). Azotemia is the accumulation of urea, creatinine and other nitrogen containing end products into the bloodstream. The regulation of fluid volume, electrolyte balance and acid base balance is also affected. The causes of acute kidney injury are divided into pre-renal (caused by a decrease in perfusion), intrarenal or intrinsic (occurring within the kidney) and post-renal (caused by the inadequate drainage of urine). Acute kidney injury is common in hospitalized patients and even more common in critically ill patients, carrying a mortality rate of 50-80%. Risk factors for acute kidney injury include advanced age, the presence of co-morbid conditions, pre-existing kidney disease and a diagnosis of sepsis.

Signs and symptoms: Malaise, fatigue, lethargy, confusion, weakness, change in urine color, change in urine volume, and flank pain.

Diagnosis: Urinalysis, serum BUN and creatinine levels, renal ultrasound, CT or MRI and renal biopsy.

Treatment: The treatment of acute kidney injury is based on the underlying cause. Treatment options may include fluid and electrolyte replacement, diuretic therapy, fluid restriction, renal diet, and low dose dopamine to increase renal perfusion. Hemodialysis may also be necessary in patients with acute kidney injury.

CHRONIC KIDNEY DISEASE

Chronic kidney disease (CKD) occurs when the kidneys are unable to filter and excrete wastes, concentrate urine, and maintain electrolyte balance because of hypoxic conditions, kidney disease, or obstruction in the urinary tract. It results first in azotemia (increase in nitrogenous waste in the blood) and then in uremia (nitrogenous wastes cause toxic symptoms.) When >50% of the functional renal capacity is destroyed, the kidneys can no longer carry out necessary functions and progressive deterioration begins over months or years. Symptoms are often non-specific in the beginning with loss of appetite and energy.

Symptoms and complications are as follows:

- Weight loss
- Headaches, muscle cramping, general malaise
- Increased bruising and dry or itchy skin
- Increased BUN and creatinine
- Sodium and fluid retention with edema
- Hyperkalemia
- Metabolic acidosis
- Calcium and phosphorus depletion, resulting in altered bone metabolism, pain, and retarded growth
- Anemia with decreased production on RBCs. Increased risk of infection
- Uremic syndrome

Treatment includes:

- Supportive/symptomatic therapy
- Dialysis and transplantation
- Diet control: Low protein, salt, potassium, and phosphorus
- Fluid limitations
- Calcium and vitamin supplementation
- Phosphate binders

Uremic Syndrome

Uremic syndrome is a number of disorders that can occur with end-stage renal disease and renal failure, usually after multiple metabolic failures and decrease in creatinine clearance to <10 mL/min. There is compromise of all normal functions of the kidney: fluid balance, electrolyte balance, acid-base homeostasis, hormone production, and elimination of wastes. Metabolic abnormalities related to uremia include:

- **Decreased RBC production:** The kidney is unable to produce adequate erythropoietin in the peritubular cells, resulting in anemia, which is usually normocytic and normochromic. Parathyroid hormone levels may increase, causing calcification of the bone marrow, causing hypoproliferative anemia as RBC production is suppressed.
- **Platelet abnormalities:** Decreased platelet count, increased turnover, and reduced adhesion leads to bleeding disorders.
- **Metabolic acidosis:** The tubular cells are unable to regulate acid-base metabolism, and phosphate, sulfuric, hippuric, and lactic acids increase, leading to congestive heart failure and weakness.
- **Hyperkalemia:** The nephrons cannot excrete adequate amounts of potassium. Some drugs, such as diuretics that spare potassium may aggravate the condition.
- **Renal bone disease:** ↓ Calcium, ↑ phosphate, ↑ parathyroid hormone, ↓ utilization of vitamin D lead to demineralization. In some cases, calcium and phosphate are deposited in other tissues (metastatic calcification).
- **Multiple endocrine disorders:** Thyroid hormone production is decreased and abnormalities in reproductive hormones may result in infertility/impotence. Males have ↓ testosterone but ↑ estrogen and LH. Females experience irregular cycles, lack of ovulation and menses. Insulin production may increase but with decreased clearance, resulting in episodes of hypoglycemia or decreased hyperglycemia in those who are diabetic.
- **Cardiovascular disorders:** Left ventricular hypertrophy is most common, but fluid retention may cause congestive heart failure and electrolyte imbalances, dysrhythmias. Pericarditis, exacerbation of valvular disorders, and pericardial effusions may occur.
- **Anorexia and malnutrition:** Nausea and poor appetite contribute to hypoalbuminemia, sometimes exacerbated by restrictive diets.

Pyelonephritis

Pyelonephritis is a potentially organ-damaging bacterial infection of the parenchyma of the kidney. Pyelonephritis can result in abscess formation, sepsis, and kidney failure. Pyelonephritis is especially dangerous for those who are immunocompromised, pregnant, or diabetic. Most infections are caused by *Escherichia coli*. **Diagnostic studies** include urinalysis, blood and urine cultures. Patients may require hospitalization or careful follow-up.

Symptoms vary widely but can include:

- Dysuria and frequency, hematuria, flank and/or low back pain
- Fever and chills
- Costovertebral angle tenderness
- Change in feeding habits (infants)
- Change in mental status (geriatric)
- Young women often exhibit symptoms more associated with lower urinary infection, so the condition may be overlooked.

Treatment includes:

- Analgesia
- Antipyretics
- Intravenous fluids
- Antibiotics: started but may be changed based on cultures
    - IV ceftriaxone with fluoroquinolone orally for 14 days
    - Monitor BUN. Normal 7-8 mg/dL (8-20 mg/dL >age 60). Increase indicates impaired renal function, as urea is end product of protein metabolism.

CYSTITIS

Cystitis is a common and often-chronic low-grade kidney infection that develops over time, so observing for symptoms of urinary infections and treating promptly are very important.

Changes in **character of urine**:

- **Appearance**: The urine may become cloudy from mucus or purulent material. Hematuria may be present.
- **Color**: Urine usually becomes concentrated and may be dark yellow/orange or brownish in color.
- **Odor**: Urine may have a very strong or foul odor.
- **Output**: Urinary output may decrease markedly.

Pain: There may be lower back or flank pain from inflammation of the kidneys.

Systemic: Fever, chills, headache, and general malaise often accompany urine infections. Some people suffer a lack of appetite as well as nausea and vomiting. Fever usually indicates that the infection has affected the kidneys. Children may develop incontinence or loose stools and cry excessively.

Treatment:

- Increased fluid intake
- Antibiotics

EPIDIDYMITIS AND ORCHITIS

Epididymitis, infection of the epididymis, is often associated with infection in a testis (epididymo-orchitis). In children, infection may be related to congenital anomalies that allow reflux of urine. In sexually active males 35 years or younger, it is usually related to STDs. In men older than 40, it is often related to urinary infections or benign prostatic hypertrophy with urethral obstruction.

Symptoms include progressive pain in lower abdomen, scrotum, and/or testicle. Late symptoms include large tender scrotal mass.

Diagnosis includes: Clinical examination. Pyuria. Urethral culture for STDs. Sonography.

Orchitis alone is rare but occurs with mumps, other viral infections, and epididymitis. Ultrasound may be needed to rule out testicular torsion.

Treatment for both conditions depends upon the cause, but epididymitis usually resolves with antibiotics:

- Younger than 40, associated with STDs:
    - Ceftriaxone 250 mg IM and doxycycline 100 mg twice daily for 10 days
- Older than 35, associated with other bacteria:
    - Ciprofloxacin 500 mg twice daily for 10-14 days
    - Levofloxacin 250 mg daily for 10-14 days
    - TMP/SMS DS twice daily for 10-14 days

PROSTATITIS

Prostatitis is an acute infection of the prostate gland, commonly caused by *Escherichia coli, Pseudomonas aeruginosa, Staphylococcus aureus,* or other bacteria. *Symptoms* include fever, chills, lower back pain, urinary frequency, dysuria, painful ejaculation, and perineal discomfort. PSA will often be elevated in this patient population, unrelated to prostate cancer. *Diagnosis* is based on clinical findings of perineal tenderness and spasm of rectal sphincter. *Treatments* include Ciprofloxacin 500 mg orally twice daily for 1 month **or** TMP/SMX DS twice daily for 1 month. Most patients also have a urethral culture to check for STDs. Patients with suspected bacteremia should be admitted for monitoring.

BENIGN PROSTATIC HYPERTROPHY

Benign prostatic hypertrophy/hyperplasia usually develops after age 40. The prostate may slowly enlarge, but the surrounding tissue restrains outward growth, so the gland compresses the urethra. The bladder wall also goes through changes, becoming thicker and irritated, so that it begins to spasm, causing frequent urinations. The bladder muscle eventually weakens and the bladder fails to empty completely.

Symptoms include urgency, dribbling, frequency, nocturia, incontinence, retention, and bladder distention.

Diagnosis may include IVP, cystogram, and PSA.

Treatment includes: Catheterization for urinary retention/bladder distention. Surgical excision. Avoid fluids close to bedtime, double void, avoid caffeine and alcohol, alpha-adrenergic antagonists, and 5-alpha-reductase inhibitors.

PID

Pelvic inflammatory disease (PID) comprises infections of the upper reproductive system, often ascending from vagina and cervix, and includes salpingitis, endometritis, tubo-ovarian abscess, peritonitis, and perihepatitis. *Neisseria gonorrhoeae* and *Chlamydia trachomatis* are implicated in most cases but some infections are polymicrobial. Complications include increase in ectopic pregnancy and tubal factor infertility. *Symptoms* include lower abdominal pain, vaginal pain, discharge, or bleeding, dyspareunia, dysuria, fever, and nausea and vomiting.

Diagnostic studies include:

- Pregnancy test
- Vaginal secretion testing, endocervical culture
- CBC
- Syphilis, HIV, and hepatitis testing

- Transvaginal pelvic ultrasound
- Endometrial biopsy
- Laparoscopy for definitive diagnosis

Treatments include:

- Broad spectrum antibiotics:
    - (Inpatient) Cefotetan 2 g IV every 12 hours or every 6 hours with doxycycline 100 mg every 12 hours
    - (Outpatient) Ceftriaxone 250 mg IM x 1 dose with doxycycline 100 mg orally every 12 hours for 14 days with metronidazole 500 mg twice daily for 2 weeks for patients who had gynecological procedures recently
- Laparoscopy to drain abscesses if symptoms do not improve in 72 hours or less
- Treatment specific to associated disorders (such as HIV or hepatitis)

Genitourinary Procedures and Interventions

PROCEDURES FOR INSERTION AND REMOVAL OF URINARY CATHETER

Procedure for inserting and removing a urinary catheter:

1. Gather supplies (included in a urinary catheter insertion kit), perform hand hygiene, place a waterproof pad under the patient, and ensure that the light source is adequate to view the urinary meatus.
2. Place females in supine position with knees flexed and males in supine position.
3. Apply gloves and wash the perineal area with facility provided cleanser (sometimes included in the outside of the urinary catheter kit) and allow to dry.
4. Remove gloves and wash hands.
5. Using aseptic technique, place the catheter kit between the patient's legs, open the kit touching only the corners of the drape that wraps around the kit.
6. Apply sterile gloves.
7. Apply sterile drapes to the patient.
8. Following the steps provided with the kit, place the lubricant into the appropriate section of tray, remove the catheter from its plastic and place the tip into the lubricant, and pour iodine over the three cleansing swabs (if they do not come impregnated with iodine already). Attach the 10-cc syringe (filled with sterile water) to the appropriate port of the catheter.
9. Cleanse the urethral meatus with the iodine impregnated swabs.
10. Using the nondominant hand, hold the penis or open the labia to observe the urethral meatus. This hand now becomes "dirty" and cannot be used to touch the catheter.
11. Using the dominant hand, insert catheter with the drainage end attached to the collection bag. Insert until urine flows freely, advancing a little further after that point.
12. Inflate the balloon using the 10-cc sterile water syringe, and ensure the catheter is secure.
13. Secure the catheter to the patient's leg and hang the collection bag below the level of the patient. Secure any tubing to the bed and ensure no kinking is present.

Removal: Straight catheter—remove by pulling out slowly. To remove indwelling catheter, deflate the balloon using the appropriate port and gently pull the catheter out.

Renal Dialysis
Peritoneal Dialysis

Renal dialysis is used primarily for those who have progressed from renal insufficiency to uremia with end-stage renal disease (ESRD). It may also be temporarily for acute conditions. People can be maintained on dialysis, but there are many complications associated with dialysis, so many people are considered for renal transplantation. There are a number of different approaches to **peritoneal dialysis:**

- **Peritoneal dialysis:** An indwelling catheter is inserted surgically into the peritoneal cavity with a subcutaneous tunnel and a Dacron cuff to prevent infection. Sterile dialysate solution is slowly instilled through gravity, remains for a prescribed length of time, and is then drained and discarded.
- **Continuous ambulatory peritoneal dialysis:** A series of exchange cycles is repeated 24 hours a day.
- **Continuous cyclic peritoneal dialysis:** A prolonged period of retaining fluid occurs during the day with drainage at night.

Peritoneal dialysis may be used for those who want to be more independent, don't live near a dialysis center, or want fewer dietary restrictions.

Hemodialysis

Hemodialysis, the most common type of dialysis, is used for both short-term dialysis and long-term for those with ESRD. Treatments are usually done 3 times weekly for 3-4 hours or daily dialysis with treatment either during the night or in short daily periods. **Hemodialysis** is often done for those who can't manage peritoneal dialysis or who live near a dialysis center, but it does interfere with work or school attendance and requires strict dietary and fluid restrictions between treatments. Short daily dialysis allows more independence, and increased costs may be offset by lower morbidity. A vascular access device, such as a catheter, fistula, or graft, must be established for hemodialysis, and heparin is used to prevent clotting. With hemodialysis, blood is circulated outside of the body through a dialyzer (a synthetic semipermeable membrane), which filters the blood. There are many different types of dialyzers. High flux dialyzers use a highly permeable membrane that shortens the duration of treatment and decreases the need for heparin.

Continuous Renal Replacement Therapy

Continuous renal replacement therapy (CRRT) circulates the blood by hydrostatic pressure through a semipermeable membrane. It is used in critical care and can be instituted quickly:

- **Continuous arteriovenous hemofiltration** (CAVH) circulates blood from an artery (usually the femoral) to a hemofilter using only arterial pressure and not a blood pump. The filtered blood is then returned to the patient's venous system, often with added fluids to offset those lost. Only the fluid is filtered.
- **Continuous arteriovenous hemodialysis** (CAVHD) is similar to CAVH except that dialysate circulates on one side of the semipermeable membrane to increase the clearance of urea.
- **Continuous venovenous hemofiltration** (CVVH) pumps blood through a double-lumen venous catheter to a hemofilter, which returns the blood to the patient in the same catheter. It provides continuous slow removal of fluid, is better tolerated with unstable patients, and doesn't require arterial access.
- **Continuous venovenous hemodialysis** is similar to CVVH but uses a dialysate to increase the clearance of uremic toxins.

Dialysis Complications

There are many complications associated with dialysis, especially when used for long-term treatment:

- **Hemodialysis**: Long-term use promotes atherosclerosis and cardiovascular disease. Anemia and fatigue are common, as are infections related to access devices or contamination of equipment. Some experience hypotension and muscle cramping during treatment. Dysrhythmias may occur. Some may exhibit dialysis disequilibrium from cerebral fluid shifts, causing headaches, nausea and vomiting, and alterations of consciousness.
- **Peritoneal dialysis:** Most complications are minor, but it can lead to peritonitis, which requires removal of the catheter if antibiotic therapy is not successful in clearing the infection within 4 days. There may be leakage of the dialysate around the catheter. Bleeding may occur, especially in females who are menstruating as blood is pulled from the uterus through the fallopian tubes. Abdominal hernias may occur with long use. Some may have anorexia from the feeling of fullness or a sweet taste in the mouth from the absorption of glucose.

Radical Nephrectomy

Radical nephrectomy is done for adenocarcinoma of the kidney, which may be associated with paraneoplastic syndromes, and, because this type of cancer is associated with smoking, patients may have underlying coronary artery or respiratory disease. Some patients have erythrocytosis, but many are anemic and may require transfusions in preparation for surgery to increase hemoglobin to >10 g/dL. Surgery is done under endotracheal general anesthesia with an anterior subcostal, flank, or thoracoabdominal (preferred for large tumors) incision. The kidney and its adrenal gland with surrounding fat and fascia are removed together. Blood loss may be extensive because the tumors tend to be vascular and large, requiring multiple transfusions. However, controlled hypotension should be limited to brief periods because it may impair renal function. Mannitol is given prior to dissection. Continual direct arterial pressure monitoring and central venous cannulation must be done.

Nephron-sparing surgery (partial nephrectomy), often by laparoscopy, may be done if the renal cell carcinoma is <4 cm diameter. Postoperative analgesia and pulmonary hygiene are essential.

Reducing Infection Risks Associated with Urinary Catheters

Strategies for reducing infection risks associated with urinary catheters include:

- Using **aseptic technique** for both the straight and indwelling catheter insertion
- **Limiting catheter use** by establishing protocols for use, duration, and removal; training staff; issuing reminders to physicians; using straight catheterizations rather than indwelling; using ultrasound to scan the bladder; and using condom catheters
- Utilizing **closed-drainage systems** for indwelling catheters
- **Avoiding irrigation** unless required for diagnosis or treatment
- Using **sampling port** for specimens rather than disconnecting catheter and tubing
- Maintaining **proper urinary flow** by proper positioning, securing of tubing and drainage bag, and keeping the drainage bag below the level of the bladder
- **Changing catheters** only when medically needed

- **Cleansing external meatal area** gently each day, manipulating the catheter as little as possible
- Avoiding placing catheterized patients adjacent to those infected or colonized with antibiotic-resistant bacteria to reduce **cross-contamination**

Bowel and Bladder Training

BLADDER TRAINING

Bladder training usually requires the person to keep a toileting diary for at least 3 days so patterns can be assessed. There are a number of different approaches:

- **Scheduled toileting** is toileting on a regular schedule, usually every 2 to 4 hours during the daytime.
- **Habit training** involves an attempt to match the scheduled toileting to a person's individual voiding habits, based on the toileting diary. This is useful for people who have a natural and fairly consistent voiding pattern. Toileting is done every 2-4 hours.
- **Prompted voiding** is often used in nursing homes and attempts to teach people to assess their own incontinence status and prompts them to ask for toileting.
- **Bladder retraining** is a behavioral modification program that teaches people to inhibit the urge to urinate and to urinate according to an established schedule, restoring normal bladder function as much as possible. Bladder training can improve incontinence in 80% of cases.

PROMPTED VOIDING

Prompted voiding is a communication protocol for people with mild to moderate **cognitive impairment**. It uses positive reinforcement for recognizing being wet or dry, staying dry, urinating, and drinking liquids.

- Ask patient **every 2 hours** (8 AM to 4-8 PM) whether they are wet or dry.
- Verify if they are correct and give **feedback**, "You are right, Mrs. Brown, you are dry."
- **Prompt** patient, whether wet or dry, to use the toilet or urinal. If yes, assist them, record results, and give positive reinforcement by praising and visiting for a short time. If no, repeat the request again once or twice. If they are wet, and decline toileting, change and tell them you will return in 2 hours and ask them to try to wait to urinate until then.
- Offer **liquids** and record amount.
- **Record** results of each attempt to urinate or wet check.

BLADDER RETRAINING

Bladder retraining teaches people to control the urge to urinate. It usually takes about 3 months to rehabilitate a bladder muscle weakened from frequent urination, causing a decreased urinary capacity. A short urination interval is gradually lengthened to every 2-4 hours during the daytime as the person suppresses bladder urges and stays dry.

- The patient keeps **urination diary** for a week.
- An individual program is established with **scheduled voiding times and goals**. For example, if a patient is urinating every hour, the goal might be every 80 minutes with increased output.

- The patient is taught **techniques** to withhold urination such as sitting on a hard seat or on a tightly rolled towel to put pressure on pelvic floor muscles, doing 5 squeezes of pelvic floor muscles, deep breathing, counting backward from 50.
- When the patient consistently meets the goal, a **new goal** is established.
- The patient keeps a **urination diary**.

THE KNACK TO CONTROL URINARY INCONTINENCE

The **knack** is the use of precisely timed muscle contractions to prevent **stress incontinence**. It is "the knack" of squeezing up before bearing down. The knack is a preventive use of **Kegel exercises**. Women are taught to contract the pelvic floor muscles right before and during events that usually cause stress incontinence. For example, if a woman feels a cough or sneeze coming, she immediately contracts the pelvic floor muscles and holds until the stress event is over. This contraction augments support of the proximal urethra, reducing the amount of displacement that usually takes place with compromised muscle support, thereby preventing incontinence. It is particularly useful if used before and during stress events, such as coughing, sneezing, lifting, standing, swinging a golf club, or laughing. Studies have shown that women who are taught this technique for mild to moderate urinary incontinence and use it consistently are able to decrease incontinence by 73-98%.

BOWEL TRAINING

Bowel training for defecation includes keeping a bowel diary to chart progress:

- **Scheduled defecation** is usually daily, but for some people 3-4 times weekly, depending on individual bowel habits. Defecation should be at the same time, so work hours and activities must be considered. Defecation is scheduled for 20-30 minutes after a meal when there is increased motility.
- **Stimulation** is necessary. Drinking a cup of hot liquid may work, but initially many require rectal stimulation, inserting a gloved, lubricated finger into the anus and running it around the rim of the sphincters. Some people require rectal suppositories, such as glycerine. Stimulus suppositories, such as Dulcolax® (bisacodyl), or even Fleet® enemas are sometimes used, but the goal is to reduce use of medical or chemical stimulants.
- **Position** should be sitting upright with knees elevated slightly if possible and leaning forward during defecation.
- **Straining** includes attempting to tighten abdominal muscles and relax sphincters while defecating.
- **Exercise** increases the motility of the bowel by stimulating muscle contractions. **Walking** is one of the best exercises for this purpose, and the person should try to walk 1 or 2 miles a day. If the person is unable to walk, then other activities, such as chair exercises that involve the arms and legs and bending can be very effective. Those who are bed bound need to turn from side to side frequently and change position.
- **Kegel exercises** increase strength of the pelvic floor muscles. Kegel exercises for urinary incontinence and fecal incontinence are essentially the same, but the person tries to pull in the muscles around the anus, as though trying to prevent the release of stool or flatus. The person should feel the muscles tightening while holding for 2 seconds and then relaxing for 2 seconds, gradually building the holding time to 10 seconds or more. Exercises should be done 4 times a day.

MANAGEMENT STRATEGIES FOR CONSTIPATION AND FECAL IMPACTION

Management strategies for constipation and impaction include:

- **Enemas** and **manual removal of impaction** may be necessary initially.
- Add **fiber** with bran, fresh/dried fruits, and whole grains, to 20-35 grams per day.
- Increase **fluids** to 64 ounces each day.
- **Exercise** program should include walking if possible, and exercises on a daily basis.
- Change in **medications** causing constipation can relieve constipation. Additionally, the use of stool softeners, such as Colace® (docusate), or bulk formers, such as Metamucil® (psyllium), may decrease fluid absorption and move stool through the colon more quickly. Overuse of laxatives can cause constipation.
- Careful **monitoring** of diet, fluids, and medical treatment, especially for irritable bowel syndrome.
- **Pregnancy-related constipation** may be controlled through dietary and fluid modifications and regular exercise.
- **Delayed toileting** should be avoided and bowel training regimen done to promote evacuation at the same time each day. During travel, stool softeners, increased fluid, and exercise may alleviate constipation.

PURPOSE OF FIBER IN THE DIET

Most constipation is caused by insufficient **fiber** in the diet, especially if people eat a lot of processed foods. An adequate amount of fiber is 20-30 grams daily. There are both soluble and insoluble forms of fiber, and both add bulk to the stool and are not absorbed into the body. Some foods have both types:

- **Soluble fiber** dissolves in liquids to form a gel-like substance, which is why liquids are so important in conjunction with fiber in the diet. Soluble fiber slows the movement of stool through the gastrointestinal system. Food sources include bananas, potatoes, dried beans, nuts, apples, oranges, and oatmeal.
- **Insoluble fiber** changes little with the digestive process and increases the speed of stool through the colon, so too much can result in diarrhea. Food sources of insoluble fiber include wheat bran, whole grains, seeds, skins of fruits, vegetables, and nuts.

Neurological Pathophysiology

NEUROLOGIC INFECTIOUS DISEASE

BACTERIAL MENINGITIS

Bacterial meningitis may be caused by a wide range of bacteria, including *Streptococcus pneumoniae* and *Neisseria meningitidis*. Bacteria can enter the CNS from distant infection, surgical wounds, invasive devices, nasal colonization, or penetrating trauma. The infective process includes inflammation, exudates, WBC accumulation, and brain tissue damage with hyperemia and edema. Purulent exudate covers the brain and invades and blocks the ventricles, obstructing CSF and leading to increased intracranial pressure. **Symptoms** include abrupt onset, fever, chills, severe headache, nuchal rigidity, and alterations of consciousness with seizures, agitation, and irritability. Antibodies specific to bacteria don't cross the blood brain barrier, so immune response is poor. Some may have photophobia, hallucinations, and/or aggressive behavior or may become stuporous and lapse into coma. Nuchal rigidity may progress to opisthotonos. Reflexes are variable but Kernig and Brudzinski signs are often positive. Signs may relate to particular bacteria, such as rashes, sore joints, or a draining ear. **Diagnosis** is usually based on lumbar puncture examination of cerebrospinal fluid and symptoms. **Treatment** includes IV antibiotics and supportive care: fluids, a dark and calm environment, measures to reduce ICP, etc.

FUNGAL MENINGITIS

Fungal meningitis is the least common cause of meningitis. It occurs when a fungal organism enters into the subarachnoid space, cerebral spinal fluid, and meninges. Immune deficient patients such as those with HIV, cancer, or immunodeficiency syndromes are most at risk for the development of fungal meningitis. The most common organisms causing fungal meningitis are candida albicans and Cryptococcus neoformans. Fungal meningitis caused by candida may occur in immunosuppressed patients, in those who have had a ventricular shunt placed, or in those that have had a lumbar puncture performed. Cryptococcus is a fungus found in soil throughout the world and does not usually affect people with a healthy immune system. Cryptococcal meningitis is most commonly seen in patients with HIV/AIDS and is one of the leading causes of death in HIV/AIDS patients in certain parts of Africa.

Signs and symptoms: Headache, fever, nausea and vomiting, stiff neck, photophobia, and mental status changes.

Diagnosis: Lumbar puncture with subsequent culture of cerebral spinal fluid. In addition, blood cultures may be obtained as well as a CT of the head.

Treatment: The treatment of fungal meningitis involves a long course of anti-fungal medications, including Amphotericin B, flucytosine, and fluconazole. Anticonvulsants may be administered for seizure control.

VIRAL INFECTIONS THAT CAN IMPACT THE NEUROLOGICAL SYSTEM

Many different types of viral infections can impact the neurological system either by direct infection transmitted through the bloodstream or by spreading along the nerve pathways (such as rabies). Common viral infections affecting the neurological system include:

- **Viral encephalitis**: Arboviral infections are transmitted from an animal host to an arthropod (typically a mosquito or tick) to humans, who are typically dead-end hosts. Arboviral infections include western equine encephalitis, eastern equine encephalitis, St. Louis encephalitis, Powassan encephalitis, Colorado tick fever and La Crosse encephalitis. West Nile virus may also invade the CNS and cause encephalitis.
- **Viral meningitis**: Viral meningitis is usually self-limiting within 7 to 10 days and is less severe than bacterial meningitis.
- **Herpes virus**: Herpes simplex virus can invade the nervous system and cause herpes simplex encephalitis, which has a high mortality rate.
- **HIV**: Inflammation may affect the CNS and interfere with neuronal functions.

NEUROMUSCULAR DISORDERS
MULTIPLE SCLEROSIS

Multiple sclerosis is an autoimmune disorder of the CNS in which the myelin sheath around the nerves is damaged and replaced by scar tissue that prevents conduction of nerve impulses.

Symptoms vary widely and can include problems with balance and coordination, tremors, slurring of speech, cognitive impairment, vision impairment, nystagmus, pain, and bladder and bowel dysfunction. Symptoms may be relapsing-remitting, progressive, or a combination. Onset is usually at 20-30 years of age, with incidence higher in females. Patient may initially present with problems walking or falling or optic neuritis (30%) causing loss of central vision. Males may complain of sexual dysfunction as an early symptom. Others have dysuria with urinary retention.

Diagnosis is based on clinical and neurological examination and MRI. **Treatment** is symptomatic and includes treatment to shorten duration of episodes and slow progress.

- **Glucocorticoids**: Methylprednisolone
- **Immunomodulator**: Interferon beta, glatiramer acetate, natalizumab
- **Immunosuppressant**: Mitoxantrone
- **Hormone**: Estriol (for females)

> **Review Video: Multiple Sclerosis**
> Visit mometrix.com/academy and enter code: 417355

ALS

Amyotrophic lateral sclerosis (ALS) is a progressive degenerative disease of the upper and lower motor neurons, resulting in progressively severe symptoms such as spasticity, hyperreflexia, muscle weakness, and paralysis that can cause dysphagia, cramping, muscular atrophy, and respiratory dysfunction. ALS may be sporadic or familial (rare). Speech may become monotone; however, cognitive functioning usually remains intact. Eventually, patients become immobile and cannot breathe independently.

Diagnosis is based on history, electromyography, nerve conduction studies, and MRI. Treatment includes riluzole to delay progression of the disease. Patients in the ED usually have been diagnosed and have developed an acute complication, such as acute respiratory failure, aspiration pneumonia, or other trauma.

Treatment includes:

- Nebulizer treatments with bronchodilators and steroids
- Antibiotics for infection
- Mechanical ventilation

If **ventilatory assistance** is needed, it is important to determine if the patient has a living will expressing the wish to be ventilated or not or has assigned power of attorney for health matters to someone to make this decision.

PARKINSON'S DISEASE

Parkinson's disease (PD) is an extrapyramidal movement motor system disorder caused by loss of brain cells that produce dopamine. Typical symptoms include tremor of face and extremities, rigidity, bradykinesia, akinesia, poor posture, and a lack of balance and coordination causing increasing problems with mobility, talking, and swallowing. Some may suffer depression and mood changes. Tremors usually present unilaterally in an upper extremity.

Diagnosis includes:

- **Cogwheel rigidity test**: The extremity is put through passive range of motion, which causes increased muscle tone and ratchet-like movements.
- Physical and neurological exam
- Complete history to rule out drug-induced Parkinson akinesia

Treatment includes:

- Symptomatic support
- Dopaminergic therapy: Levodopa, amantadine, and carbidopa
- Anticholinergics: Trihexyphenidyl, benztropine
- For drug-induced Parkinson's, terminate drugs

Drug therapy tends to decrease in effectiveness over time, and patients may present with a marked increase in symptoms. Discontinuing the drugs for 1 week may exacerbate symptoms initially, but functioning may improve when drugs are reintroduced.

GUILLAIN-BARRÉ SYNDROME

Guillain-Barré syndrome (GBS) is an autoimmune disorder of the myelinated motor peripheral nervous system, causing ascending and descending paralysis. GBS is often triggered by a viral infection, but may be idiopathic in origin. Diagnosis is by history, clinical symptoms, and lumbar puncture, which often show increased protein with normal glucose and cell count although protein may not increase for a week or more.

> **Review Video: Guillain-Barre Syndrome**
> Visit mometrix.com/academy and enter code: 742900

Symptoms include:

- Numbness and tingling with increasing weakness of lower extremities that may become generalized, sometimes resulting in complete paralysis and inability to breathe without ventilatory support.
- Deep tendon reflexes are typically absent and some people experience facial weakness and ophthalmoplegia (paralysis of muscles controlling movement of eyes).

Treatment includes:

- Supportive: Fluids, physical therapy, and antibiotics for infections
- Patients should be hospitalized for observation and placed on ventilator support if forced vital capacity is reduced.
- While there is no definitive treatment, plasma exchange or IV immunoglobulin may shorten the duration of symptoms.

MUSCULAR DYSTROPHY

Muscular dystrophies are genetic disorders with gradual degeneration of muscle fibers and progressive weakness and atrophy of skeletal muscles and loss of mobility. **Pseudohypertrophic (Duchenne) muscular dystrophy** is the most common form and the most severe. It is an X-linked disorder in about 50% of the cases with the rest sporadic mutations, affecting males almost exclusively. Children typically have some delay in motor development with difficulty walking and have evidence of muscle weakness by about age 3. Pseudohypertrophic refers to enlargement of muscles by fatty infiltration associated with muscular atrophy, which causes contractures and deformities of joints. Abnormal bone development results in spinal and other skeletal deformities. The disease progresses rapidly, and most children are wheelchair bound by about 12 years of age. As the disease progresses, it involves the muscles of the diaphragm and other muscles needed for respiration. Mild to frank mental deficiency is common. Facial, oropharyngeal, and respiratory muscles weaken late in the disease. Cardiomegaly commonly occurs. Death most often relates to respiratory infection or cardiac failure by age 25. Treatment is supportive.

CEREBRAL PALSY

Cerebral palsy (CP) is a non-progressive motor dysfunction related to CNS damage associated with congenital, hypoxic, or traumatic injury before, during, or ≤2 years after birth. It may include visual defects, speech impairment, seizures, and mental retardation. There are four **types of motor dysfunction:**

- **Spastic**: Damage to the cerebral cortex or pyramidal tract. Constant hypertonia and rigidity lead to contractures and curvature of the spine.
- **Dyskinetic**: Damage to the extrapyramidal, basal ganglia. Tremors and twisting with exaggerated posturing and impairment of voluntary muscle control.
- **Ataxic**: Damage to the extrapyramidal cerebellum. Atonic muscles in infancy with lack of balance, instability of muscles, and poor gait.
- **Mixed**: Combinations of all three types with multiple areas of damage.

Characteristics of CP include:

- Hypotonia or hypertonia with rigidity and spasticity
- Athetosis (constant writhing motions)
- Ataxia
- Hemiplegia (one-sided involvement, more severe in upper extremities)
- Diplegia (all extremities involved, but more severe in lower extremities)
- Quadriplegia (all extremities involved with arms flexed and legs extended)

MYASTHENIA GRAVIS

Myasthenia gravis is an autoimmune disorder that results in sporadic, progressive weakness of striated (skeletal) muscles because of impaired transmission of nerve impulses. Myasthenia gravis usually affects muscles controlled by the cranial nerves although any muscle group may be affected. Many patients also have thymomas.

Signs and symptoms include weakness and fatigue that worsens throughout the day. Patients often exhibit ptosis and diplopia. They may have trouble chewing and swallowing and often appear to have masklike facies. If respiratory muscles are involved, patients may exhibit signs of respiratory failure. Myasthenic crisis occurs when patients can no longer breathe independently.

Diagnosis includes electromyography and the Tensilon test (an IV injection of edrophonium or neostigmine, which improves function if the patient has myasthenia gravis, but does not improve function if the symptoms are from a different cause). CT or MRI to diagnose thymoma.

Treatment includes anticholinesterase drugs (neostigmine, pyridostigmine) to relieve some muscle weakness, but these drugs lose effectiveness as the disease progresses. Corticosteroids may be used. Thymectomy is performed if thymoma is present. Tracheotomy and mechanical ventilation may be needed for myasthenic crisis.

Seizure Disorders
Partial Seizures
Partial seizures are caused by electrical discharges to a localized area of the cerebral cortex, such as the frontals, temporal, or parietal lobes with seizure characteristics related to the area of involvement. They may begin in a focal area and become generalized, often preceded by an aura.

- **Simple partial:** Unilateral motor symptoms including somatosensory, psychic, and autonomic
  - Aversive: Eyes and head turned away from focal side
  - Sylvan (usually during sleep): Tonic-clonic movements of the face, salivation, and arrested speech
- **Special sensory:** Various sensations (numbness, tingling, prickling, or pain) spreading from one area. May include visual sensations, posturing or hypertonia.
- **Complex (Psychomotor):** No loss of consciousness, but altered consciousness and non-responsive with amnesia. May involve complex sensorium with bad tastes, auditory or visual hallucinations, feeling of déjà vu, strong fear. May carry out repetitive activities, such as walking, running, smacking lips, chewing, or drawling. Rarely aggressive. Seizure usually followed by prolonged drowsiness and confusion. Most common ages 3 through adolescence.

Generalized Seizures
Generalized seizures lack a focal onset and appear to involve both hemispheres, usually presenting with loss of consciousness and no preceding aura.

- **Tonic-clonic (Grand Mal):** Occurs without warning
  - Tonic period (10-30 seconds): Eyes roll upward with loss of consciousness, arms flexed; stiffen in symmetric tonic contraction of body, apneic with cyanosis and salivating
  - Clonic period (10 seconds to 30 minutes, but usually 30 seconds). Violent rhythmic jerking with contraction and relaxation. May be incontinent of urine and feces. Contractions slow and then stop.

Following seizures, there may be confusion, disorientation, and impairment of motor activity, speech, and vision for several hours. Headache, nausea, and vomiting may occur. Person often falls asleep and awakens more lucid.

- **Absence (Petit Mal):** Onset is at ages 4-12 and usually ends in puberty. Onset is abrupt with brief loss of consciousness for 5-10 seconds and slight loss of muscle tone but often appears to be daydreaming. Lip smacking or eye twitching may occur.

Epilepsy
Epilepsy is diagnosed based on a history of seizure activity as well as supporting EEG findings. Treatment is individualized. First line treatments include antiepileptic medications for partial and generalized tonic-clonic seizures. Usually, treatment is started with one medication, but this may need to be changed, adjusted, or an additional medication added until the seizures are under control or to avoid adverse effects, which include allergic reactions, especially skin irritations and acute or chronic toxicity. Milder reactions often subside with time or adjustment in doses. Toxic reactions may vary considerably, depending upon the medication and duration of use, so close monitoring is essential. Severe rash and hepatotoxicity are common toxic reactions that occur with many of the antiepileptic drugs. Dosages of drugs may need to be adjusted to avoid breakthrough

seizures during times of stress, such as during illness or surgery. Alcohol/drug abuse and sleep deprivation may also cause breakthrough seizures. Most anticonvulsant drugs are teratogenic.

STATUS EPILEPTICUS

Status epilepticus (SE) is usually generalized tonic-clonic seizures that are characterized by a series of seizures with intervening time too short for regaining of consciousness. The constant assault and periods of apnea can lead to exhaustion, respiratory failure with hypoxemia and hypercapnia, cardiac failure, and death.

Causes: Uncontrolled epilepsy or non-compliance with anticonvulsants, infections such as encephalitis, encephalopathy or stroke, drug toxicity (isoniazid), brain trauma, neoplasms, and metabolic disorders.

Treatment includes:

- Anticonvulsants usually beginning with a fast-acting benzodiazepine (lorazepam), often in steps, with administration of medication every 5 minutes until seizures subside.
- If cause is undetermined, acyclovir and ceftriaxone may be administered.
- If there is no response to the first 2 doses of anticonvulsants (refractory SE), rapid sequence intubation (RSI), which involves sedation and paralytic anesthesia, may be done while therapy continues. Combining phenobarbital and benzodiazepine can cause apnea, so intubation may be necessary.
- Antiepileptic medications are added.

BRAIN TUMORS

Any type of brain tumor can occur in adults. Brain tumors may be primary, arising within the brain, or secondary as a result of metastasis:

- **Astrocytoma**: This arises from astrocytes, which are glial cells. It is the most common type of tumor, occurring throughout the brain. There are many types of astrocytomas, and most are slow growing. Some are operable while others are not. Radiation may be given after removal. Astrocytomas include glioblastomas, aggressively malignant tumors occurring most often in adults 45-70.
- **Glioblastoma**: This is the most common and most malignant adult brain tumor/astrocytoma. Treatment includes surgery, radiation, and chemotherapy, but survival rates are very low.
- **Brain stem glioma**: This may be fast or slow growing but is generally not operable because of location, although it may be treated with radiation or chemotherapy.
- **Craniopharyngioma**: This is a congenital, slow-growing, recurrent (especially if >5 cm) and benign cystic tumor that is difficult to resect and is treated with surgery and radiation.
- **Meningioma**: Slow growing recurrent tumors are usually benign and most often occur in women, ages 40-70; however, they can cause severe impairment/death, depending on size and location. Meningiomas are surgically removed if causing symptoms.
- **Ganglioglioma**: This can occur anywhere in the brain and is usually slow growing and benign.
- **Medulloblastoma**: There are many types of medulloblastoma, most arising in the cerebellum, malignant, and fast growing. Surgical excision is often followed by radiation and chemotherapy although recent studies show using just chemotherapy controls recurrence with less neurological damage.

- **Oligodendroglioma**: This tumor most often occurs in the cerebrum, primarily the frontal or temporal lobes, involving the myelin sheath of the neurons. It is slow growing and most common in those age 40-60.
- **Optical nerve glioma**: This slow growing tumor of the optic nerve is usually a form of astrocytoma. Optic nerve glioma is often associated with neurofibromatosis type I (NF1), occurring in 15-40% of patients with NF1. Despite surgical, chemotherapy, or radiotherapy treatment, it is usually fatal.

STROKES
HEMORRHAGIC STROKES
Hemorrhagic strokes account for about 20% of all strokes and result from a ruptured cerebral artery, causing not only a lack of oxygen and nutrients but also edema that causes widespread pressure and damage:

- **Intracerebral** is bleeding into the substance of the brain from an artery in the central lobes, basal ganglia, pons, or cerebellum. Intracerebral hemorrhage usually results from atherosclerotic degenerative changes, hypertension, brain tumors, anticoagulation therapy, or use of illicit drugs, such as cocaine.
- **Intracranial aneurysm** occurs with ballooning cerebral artery ruptures, most commonly at the Circle of Willis.
- **Arteriovenous malformation**. Rupture of AVMs can cause brain attack in young adults.
- **Subarachnoid hemorrhage** is bleeding in the space between the meninges and brain, resulting from aneurysm, AVM, or trauma. This type of hemorrhage compresses brain tissue.

Treatment includes: The patient may need airway protection/artificial ventilation if neurologic compromise is severe. Blood pressure is lowered to control rate of bleeding but with caution to avoid hypotension and resulting cerebral ischemia (Goal – CPP >70). Sedation can lower ICP and blood pressure, and seizure prophylaxis will be indicated as blood irritates the cerebral cells. An intraventricular catheter may be used in ICP management; correct any clotting disorders if identified.

ISCHEMIA STROKES
Strokes (brain attacks, cerebrovascular accidents) result when there is interruption of the blood flow to an area of the brain. The two basic types are ischemic and hemorrhagic. About 80% are **ischemic**, resulting from blockage of an artery supplying the brain:

- **Thrombosis** in a large artery, usually resulting from atherosclerosis, may block circulation to a large area of the brain. It is most common in the elderly and may occur suddenly or after episodes of transient ischemic attacks.
- **Lacunar infarct** (a penetrating thrombosis in a small artery) is most common in those with diabetes mellitus and/or hypertension.
- **Embolism** travels through the arterial system and lodges in the brain, most commonly in the left middle cerebral artery. An embolism may be cardiogenic, resulting from cardiac arrhythmia or surgery. An embolism usually occurs rapidly with no warning signs.
- **Cryptogenic** has no identifiable cause.

Medical management of ischemic strokes with tissue plasminogen activator (tPA) (Activase®), the primary treatment, should be initiated within 3 hours (or up to 4.5 hours if inclusion criteria are met):

- **Thrombolytic,** such as tPA, which is produced by recombinant DNA and is used to dissolve fibrin clots. It is given intravenously (0.9 mg/kg up to 90 mg) with 10% injected as an initial bolus and the rest over the next hour.
- **Antihypertensives** if MAP >130 mmHg or systolic BP >220
- **Cooling** to reduce hyperthermia
- **Osmotic diuretics** (mannitol), hypertonic saline, loop diuretics (Lasix®), and/or corticosteroids (dexamethasone) to decrease cerebral edema and intracranial pressure
- **Aspirin/anticoagulation** may be used with embolism
- Monitor and treat hyperglycemia
- **Surgical Intervention:** Used when other treatment fails, may go in through artery and manually remove the clot

SYMPTOMS OF BRAIN ATTACKS IN RELATION TO AREA OF BRAIN AFFECTED

Brain attacks most commonly occur in the right or left hemisphere, but the exact location and the extent of brain damage from a brain attack affects the type of presenting symptoms. If the frontal area of either side is involved, there tends to be memory and learning deficits. Some symptoms are common to specific areas and help to identify the area involved:

- **Right hemisphere**: This results in left paralysis or paresis and a left visual field deficit that may cause spatial and perceptual disturbances, so people may have difficulty judging distance. Fine motor skills may be impacted, resulting in trouble dressing or handling tools. People may become impulsive and exhibit poor judgment, often denying impairment. Left-sided neglect (lack of perception of things on the left side) may occur. Depression is common as well as short-term memory loss and difficulty following directions. Language skills usually remain intact.
- **Left hemisphere**: Results in right paralysis or paresis and a right visual field defect. Depression is common and people often exhibit slow, cautious behavior, requiring repeated instruction and reinforcement for simple tasks. Short-term memory loss and difficulty learning new material or understanding generalizations is common. Difficulty with mathematics, reading, writing, and reasoning may occur. Aphasia (expressive, receptive, or global) is common.
- **Brain stem**: Because the brain stem controls respiration and cardiac function, a brain attack in the brain stem frequently causes death, but those who survive may have a number of problems, including respiratory and cardiac abnormalities. Strokes may involve motor or sensory impairment or both.
- **Cerebellum**: This area controls balance and coordination. Brain attacks in the cerebellum are rare but may result in ataxia, nausea and vomiting, and headaches and dizziness or vertigo.

TIA

Transient ischemic attacks (TIAs) from small clots cause similar but short-lived (minutes to hours) symptoms. Emergent treatment includes placing patient in semi-Fowlers or Fowler's position and administering oxygen. The patient may require oral suctioning if secretions pool. The patient's circulation, airway, and breathing should be assessed and IV access line placed. Thrombolytic therapy to dissolve blood clots should be administered within 1 to 3 hours. While a patient can recover fully from a TIA, they should be educated, because having a TIA increases an individual's risk for a stroke.

DELIRIUM

Delirium is an acute, sudden, and fluctuating change in consciousness. Delirium occurs in 10-40% of hospitalized older adults and about 80% of patients who are terminally ill. Delirium may result from drugs, infections, hypoxia, trauma, dementia, depression, vision and hearing loss, surgery, alcoholism, untreated pain, fluid/electrolyte imbalance, and malnutrition. If left untreated, delirium greatly increases the risk of morbidity and death.

Signs/Symptoms: Reduced ability to focus/sustain attention, language and memory disturbances, disorientation, confusion, audiovisual hallucinations, sleep disturbance, and psychomotor activity disorder.

Diagnosis: Patient interview, history/chart/medication review, and possible blood tests to identify electrolyte imbalance/abnormalities.

Treatment includes:

- **Medications**: Trazodone, lorazepam, haloperidol—though these may make confusion worse in elderly patients
- **Procedures**: Provide a sitter to ensure safety, decreasing dosage of hypnotics and psychotropics, correct underlying cause

Prevention: Reorient patient frequently, ensure adequate rest/nutrition, monitor response to medications, and treat infections and dehydration/malnutrition early.

AGITATION

Agitation is a common occurrence in the critically ill patient. Factors contributing to the development of agitation include drug or alcohol withdrawal, sleep deprivation, hypoxemia, electrolyte or metabolic imbalance, anxiety, pain, and adverse drug reactions. Delirium may also include agitation as a manifestation.

Diagnosis: The physiologic effects of agitation may include increases in heart rate, respiratory rate, blood pressure, intracranial pressure, and oxygen consumption. In addition, agitation can contribute to the self-removal of lines or tubes and combative behavior that may result in patient harm.

Treatment: Treatment of agitation involves the identification and correction of causative factors. The use of pharmacologic agents to manage pain, anxiety, and agitation are often utilized. Non-pharmacologic interventions including verbal de-escalation (when possible). The promotion of normal sleep patterns and relaxation techniques may also be effective. Early identification of signs and symptoms is also critical in the successful management of agitation.

Dementia

Dementia is a chronic condition in which there is progressive and irreversible loss of memory and function. There are many types of dementia a nurse may encounter:

1. **Creutzfeldt-Jakob disease**: Rapidly progressive dementia with impaired memory, behavioral changes, and incoordination
2. **Dementia with Lewy Bodies**: Similar to Alzheimer's, but symptoms may fluctuate frequently; may also include visual hallucinations, muscle rigidity, and tremors
3. **Frontotemporal dementia**: Causes marked changes in personality and behavior; characterized by difficulty using and understanding language
4. **Mixed dementia**: Combination of different types of dementia
5. **Normal pressure hydrocephalus**: Characterized by ataxia, memory loss, and urinary incontinence
6. **Parkinson's dementia**: Involves impaired decision making and difficulty concentrating, learning new material, understanding complex language, and sequencing
7. **Vascular dementia**: Memory loss less pronounced than that common to Alzheimer's, but symptoms are similar

Nursing considerations: Distraction is usually the best course of action to deter the patient with dementia. Reorient frequently, but do not argue with the patient. Avoid restraints or sedatives, which worsen confusion.

Respiratory Pathophysiology

Acute Lung Injury and Acute Respiratory Distress Syndrome

Acute lung injury (ALI) comprises a syndrome of respiratory distress culminating in acute respiratory distress syndrome (ARDS). ARDS is a dangerous, potentially fatal respiratory condition, always caused by an illness or injury to the lungs. Lung injury causes fluid to leak into the spaces between the alveoli and capillaries, increasing pressure on the alveoli, causing them to collapse. With increased fluid accumulation in the lungs, the ability of the lungs to move oxygen into the blood is decreased, resulting in hypoxemia. Lung injury also causes a release of cytokines, a type of inflammatory protein, which then brings neutrophils to the lung. These proteins and cells leak into nearby blood vessels and cause inflammation throughout the body. This immune response, in combination with low levels of blood oxygen, can lead to organ failure. Symptoms are characterized by respiratory distress within 72 hours of surgery or a serious injury to a person with otherwise normal lungs and no cardiac disorder. Untreated, the condition results in respiratory failure, MODS, and a mortality rate of 5-30%.

Symptoms include:

- Refractory hypoxemia (hypoxemia not responding to increasing levels of oxygen)
- Crackling rales/wheezing in lungs
- Decrease in pulmonary compliance which results in increased tachypnea with expiratory grunting
- Cyanosis/skin mottling
- Hypotension and tachycardia
- Symptoms associated with volume overload are missing (3rd heart sound or JVD)

- Respiratory alkalosis initially but, as the disease progresses, replaced with hypercarbia and respiratory acidosis
- Normal x-ray initially but then diffuse infiltrates in both lungs, while the heart and vessels appear normal

Management

The management of acute respiratory distress syndrome (ARDS) involves providing adequate gas exchange and preventing further damage to the lung from forced ventilation.

Treatment includes:

- Mechanical ventilation to maintain oxygenation and ventilation
- Corticosteroids (may increase mortality rates in some patient populations, though this is the most commonly given treatment), nitrous oxide, inhaled surfactant, and anti-inflammatory medications
- Treatment of the underlying condition is the only proven treatment, especially identifying and treating an infection with appropriate antibiotics, as sepsis is most common etiology for ARDS, but prophylactic antibiotics are not indicated.
- Conservative fluid management is indicated to reduce days on the ventilator, but does not reduce overall mortality.

Pharmacologic preventive care: Enoxaparin 40 mg subcutaneously QD, sucralfate 1 g NGT four times daily or omeprazole 40 mg IV QD, and enteral nutrition support within 24 hours of ICU admission or intubation.

Ventilation Management

Ventilation management in ARDS consists of the following:

- O_2 therapy by nasal prongs, cannula, or mask may be sufficient in very mild cases to maintain oxygen saturation above 90%. Oxygen should be administered at 100% because of the mismatch between ventilation (V) and perfusion (Q), which can result in hypoxia on position change.
- ARDS oxygenation goal is PaO_2 55-80 mmHg or SpO_2 88-95%.
- Endotracheal intubation may be needed if SpO_2 falls or CO_2 levels rise.
- The ARDS Network recommends low tidal volumes (6 mL/kg) and higher PEEP (12 cmH_2O or more).
- The low tidal volume ventilation described above is referred to as lung protective ventilation, and it has been shown to reduce mortality in patients with ARDS.
- Placing patients with severe ARDS in prone position for 18-24 hours per day with chest and pelvis supported and abdomen unsupported allows the diaphragm to move posteriorly, increasing functional residual capacity (FRC) in many patients.

Acute Respiratory Failure
Cardinal Signs

The cardinal signs of respiratory failure include:

- Tachypnea
- Tachycardia
- Anxiety and restlessness
- Diaphoresis

Symptoms may vary according to the cause. An obstruction may cause more obvious respiratory symptoms than other disorders.

- Early signs may include changes in the depth and pattern of respirations with flaring nares, sternal retractions, expiratory grunting, wheezing, and extended expiration as the body tries to compensate for hypoxemia and increasing levels of carbon dioxide.
- Cyanosis may be evident.
- Central nervous depression, with alterations in consciousness occurs with decreased perfusion to the brain.
- As the hypoxemia worsens, cardiac arrhythmias, including bradycardia, may occur with either hypotension or hypertension.
- Dyspnea becomes more pronounced with depressed respirations.
- Eventually stupor, coma, and death can occur if the condition is not reversed.

HYPOXEMIC AND HYPERCAPNIC RESPIRATORY FAILURE

Hypoxemic respiratory failure occurs suddenly when gaseous exchange of oxygen for carbon dioxide cannot keep up with demand for oxygen or production of carbon dioxide:

- PaO_2 <60 mmHg
- $PaCO_2$ >40 mmHg
- Arterial pH <7.35

Hypoxemic respiratory failure can be the result of low inhaled oxygen, as at high elevations or with smoke inhalation. The following ventilatory mechanisms may be involved:

- Alveolar hypotension
- Ventilation-perfusion mismatch (the most common cause)
- Intrapulmonary shunts
- Diffusion impairment

Hypercapnic respiratory failure results from an increase in $PaCO_2$ >45-50 mmHg associated with respiratory acidosis and may include:

- Reduction in minute ventilation, total volume of gas ventilated in one minute (often related to neurological, muscle, or chest wall disorders, drug overdoses, or obstruction of upper airway)
- Increased dead space with wasted ventilation (related to lung disease or disorders of chest wall, such as scoliosis)
- Increased production of CO_2 (usually related to infection, burns, or other causes of hypermetabolism)
- Oxygen saturation normal or below normal

UNDERLYING CAUSES

There are a number of underlying causes for respiratory failure:

- **Airway obstruction:** Obstruction may result from an inhaled object or from an underlying disease process, such as cystic fibrosis, asthma, pulmonary edema, or infection.
- **Inadequate respirations:** This is a common cause among adults, especially related to obesity and sleep apnea. It may also be induced by an overdose of sedation medications such as opioids.

- **Neuromuscular disorders:** Those disorders that interfere with the neuromuscular functioning of the lungs or the chest wall, such as muscular dystrophy or spinal cord injuries can prevent adequate ventilation.
- **Pulmonary abnormalities:** Those abnormalities of the lung tissue, found in pulmonary fibrosis, burns, ARDS, and reactions to drugs, can lead to failure.
- **Chest wall abnormalities:** Disorders that impact lung parenchyma, such as severe scoliosis or chest wounds can interfere with lung functioning.

Nursing interventions to help prevent respiratory issues:

- Turn, position, and ambulate the patient.
- Have the patient cough and breathe deeply.
- Use vibration and percussion treatments.
- Hydrate the patient to help hydrate the airway secretions, and incentive spirometry.

MANAGEMENT

Respiratory failure must be **treated** immediately before severe hypoxemia causes irreversible damage to vital organs.

- **Identifying and treating** the underlying cause should be done immediately because emergency medications or surgery may be indicated. Medical treatments will vary widely depending upon the cause; for example, cardiopulmonary structural defects may require surgical repair, pulmonary edema may require diuresis, inhaled objects may require surgical removal, and infections may require aggressive antimicrobials.
- **Intravenous lines/central lines** are inserted for testing, fluids, and medications.
- **Oxygen therapy** should be initiated to attempt to reverse hypoxemia; however, if refractory hypoxemia occurs, then oxygen therapy alone will not suffice. Oxygen levels must be titrated carefully.
- **Intubation and mechanical ventilation** are frequently required to maintain adequate ventilation and oxygenation. Positive end expiratory pressure (PEEP) may be necessary with refractory hypoxemia and collapsed alveoli.
- **Respiratory status** must be monitored constantly, including arterial blood gases and vital signs.

PNEUMONIA

Pneumonia is inflammation of the lung parenchyma, filling the alveoli with exudate. It is common throughout childhood and adulthood. Pneumonia may be a primary disease or may occur secondary to another infection or disease, such as lung cancer. Pneumonia may be caused by bacteria, viruses, parasites, or fungi. Common causes for community-acquired pneumonia (CAP) include:

- *Streptococcus pneumoniae*
- *Legionella* species
- *Haemophilus influenzae*
- *Staphylococcus aureus*
- *Mycoplasma pneumoniae*
- Viruses

Pneumonia may also be caused by chemical damage. Pneumonia is characterized by **location**:

- **Lobar** involves one or more lobes of the lungs. If lobes in both lungs are affected, it is referred to as bilateral or double pneumonia.
- **Bronchial/lobular** involves the terminal bronchioles, and exudate can involve the adjacent lobules. Usually, the pneumonia occurs in scattered patches throughout the lungs.
- **Interstitial** involves primarily the interstitium and alveoli where white blood cells and plasma fill the alveoli, generating inflammation and creating fibrotic tissue as the alveoli are destroyed.

> **Review Video: Pneumonia**
> Visit mometrix.com/academy and enter code: 628264

HOSPITAL-ACQUIRED PNEUMONIA

Hospital-acquired pneumonia (HAP) is defined as pneumonia that did not appear to be present on admission that occurs at least 48 hours after admission to a hospital. **Healthcare-associated pneumonia (HCAP)** is defined as pneumonia that occurs in a patient within 90 days of being hospitalized for 2 or more days at an acute care hospital or LTAC. **Ventilator-associated pneumonia (VAP)** is one type of hospital acquired pneumonia that a patient acquires more than 48 hours after having an ETT placed. The most common way that the patient is infected is via aspiration of bacteria that is colonized in the upper respiratory tract. It is estimated that close to 75% of patients that are critically ill will be colonized with multidrug resistant bacteria within 48 hours of entering an ICU. Aspiration occurs at a rate of about 45% in patients with no health problems and the rate is much higher in those with HAP, HCAP, and VAP. The frequency of patients developing these types of pneumonia is increasing, with those at highest risk being those with immunosuppression, septic shock, currently hospitalized for more than five days, and those who have had antibiotics for another infection within the previous three months. These types of pneumonia should be considered if a patient already hospitalized has purulent sputum or a change in respiratory status such as deoxygenating, in combination with a worsening or new chest x-ray infiltrate.

Treatment includes:

- Antibiotic therapy
- Using appropriate isolation and precautions with infected patients
- Preventive measures including maintaining ventilated patients in 30° upright positions, frequent oral care for vent patients, and changing ventilator circuits as per protocol

Antibiotic treatment options for HAP, HCAP, and VAP should take into account many factors, including culture data (when available), patient's comorbidities, flora in the unit, any recent antibiotics by the patient, and whether the patient is at high risk for having multidrug resistant bacteria. As most critical care patients are at high risk, due to factors such as being in an ICU setting, ventilators, and comorbidities, antibiotic recommendations to follow are for coverage for patients with risk factors for multidrug resistant bacteria.

One of the following:

- Ceftazidime 2 g every 8 hours IV **OR**
- Cefepime 2 g every 8 hours IV **OR**
- Imipenem 500 mg every 6 hours IV **OR**
- Piperacillin-tazobactam 4.5 g every 6 hours IV

AND one of the following:

- Ciprofloxacin 400 mg every 8 hours IV **OR**
- Levaquin 750 mg every 24 hours IV

ASPIRATION PNEUMONITIS/PNEUMONIA

Aspiration pneumonitis/pneumonia may occur as the result of any type of aspiration, including foreign objects. The aspirated material creates an inflammatory response, with the irritated mucous membrane at high risk for bacterial infection secondary to the aspiration, causing pneumonia. Gastric contents and oropharyngeal bacteria are commonly aspirated. Gastric contents can cause a severe chemical pneumonitis with hypoxemia, especially if the pH is <2.5. Acidic food particles can cause severe reactions. With acidic damage, bronchospasm and atelectasis occur rapidly with tracheal irritation, bronchitis, and alveolar damage with interstitial edema and hemorrhage. Intrapulmonary shunting and V/Q mismatch may occur. Pulmonary artery pressure increases. Non-acidic liquids and food particles are less damaging, and symptoms may clear within 4 hours of liquid aspiration or granuloma may form about food particles in 1-5 days. Depending upon the type of aspiration, pneumonitis may clear within a week, ARDS or pneumonia may develop, or progressive acute respiratory failure may lead to death.

There are a number of risk factors that can lead to **aspiration pneumonitis/pneumonia:**

- Altered level of consciousness related to illness or sedation
- Depression of gag, swallowing reflex
- Intubation or feeding tubes
- Ileus or gastric distention
- Gastrointestinal disorders, such as gastroesophageal reflux disorders (GERD)

Diagnosis is based on clinical findings, ABGs showing hypoxemia, infiltrates observed on x-ray, and ↑ WBC if infection is present.

Symptoms: Similar to other pneumonias:

- Cough often with copious sputum
- Respiratory distress, dyspnea
- Cyanosis
- Tachycardia
- Hypotension

Treatment includes:

- Suctioning as needed to clear upper airway
- Supplemental oxygen
- Antibiotic therapy as indicated after 48 hours if symptoms not resolving
- Symptomatic respiratory support

FOREIGN BODY ASPIRATION

Foreign body aspiration can cause obstruction of the pharynx, larynx, or trachea, leading to acute dyspnea or asphyxiation, and the object may also be drawn distally into the bronchial tree. With adults, most foreign bodies migrate more readily down the right bronchus. Food is the most frequently aspirated, but other small objects, such as coins or needles, may also be aspirated. Sometimes the object causes swelling, ulceration, and general inflammation that hampers removal.

Symptoms include:

- **Initial**: Severe coughing, gagging, sternal retraction, wheezing. Objects in the larynx may cause inability to breathe or speak and lead to respiratory arrest. Objects in the bronchus cause cough, dyspnea, and wheezing.
- **Delayed**: Hours, days, or weeks later, an undetected aspirant may cause an infection distal to the aspirated material. Symptoms depend on the area and extent of the infection.

Treatment includes:

- Removal with laryngoscopy or bronchoscopy (rigid is often better than flexible)
- Antibiotic therapy for secondary infection
- Surgical bronchotomy (rarely required)
- Symptomatic support

CHRONIC BRONCHITIS

Chronic bronchitis is a pulmonary airway disease characterized by severe cough with sputum production for at least 3 months a year for at least 2 consecutive years. Irritation of the airways (often from smoke or pollutants) causes an inflammatory response, increasing the number of mucus-secreting glands and goblet cells while ciliary function decreases so that the extra mucus plugs the airways. Additionally, the bronchial walls thicken, alveoli near the inflamed bronchioles become fibrotic, and alveolar macrophages cannot function properly, increasing susceptibility to infections. Chronic bronchitis is most common in those >45 years old and occurs twice as frequently in females as males.

Symptoms include:

- Persistent cough with increasing sputum
- Dyspnea
- Frequent respiratory infections

Treatment includes:

- Bronchodilators
- Long term continuous oxygen therapy or supplemental oxygen during exercise
- Pulmonary rehabilitation to improve exercise and breathing
- Antibiotics during infections
- Corticosteroids for acute episodes

EMPHYSEMA

Emphysema, the primary component of COPD, is characterized by abnormal distention of air spaces at the ends of the terminal bronchioles, with destruction of alveolar walls so that there is less and less gaseous exchange and increasing dead space with resultant hypoxemia, hypercapnia, and respiratory acidosis. The capillary bed is damaged as well, altering pulmonary blood flow and raising pressure in the right atrium (cor pulmonale) and pulmonary artery, leading to cardiac failure. Complications include respiratory insufficiency and failure. There are two primary types of emphysema (and both forms may be present):

- **Centrilobular** (the most common form) involves the central portion of the respiratory lobule, sparing distal alveoli, and usually affects the upper lobes. Typical symptoms include abnormal ventilation-perfusion ratios, hypoxemia, hypercapnia, and polycythemia with right-sided heart failure.
- **Panlobular** involves enlargement of all air spaces, including the bronchiole, alveolar duct, and alveoli, but there is minimal inflammatory disease. Typical symptoms include hyperextended rigid barrel chest, marked dyspnea, weight loss, and active expiration.

COPD

STAGES

Functional dyspnea, body mass index (BMI), and spirometry are used to assess the **stages of chronic obstructive pulmonary disease (COPD)**. Spirometry measures used are the ratio of forced expiratory volume in the first second of expiration (FEV_1) after full inhalation to total forced vital capacity (FVC). Normal lung function decreases after age 35; so normal values are adjusted for height, weight, gender, and age:

- **Stage 1** (mild): Minimal dyspnea with or without cough and sputum. FEV_1 is ≥80% of predicted rate and FEV_1:FVC <70%.
- **Stage 2** (moderate): Moderate to severe chronic exertional dyspnea with or without cough and sputum. FEV_1 is 50-80% of predicted rate and FEV_1:FVC <70%.
- **Stage 3** (severe): Same as stage 2 but with repeated episodes with increased exertional dyspnea and condition impacting quality of life. FEV_1 is 30-50% of predicted rate and FEV_1:FVC <70%.
- **Stage 4** (very severe): Severe dyspnea and life-threatening episodes that severely impact quality of life. FEV_1 is 30% of predicted rate or <50% with chronic respiratory failure and FEV_1:FVC <70%.

MANAGEMENT

COPD is not reversible, so management aims at slowing its progression, relieving symptoms, and improving quality of life:

- Smoking cessation is the primary means to slow progression and may require smoking cessation support in the form of classes or medications, such as Zyban®, nicotine patches or gum, clonidine, or nortriptyline.
- Bronchodilators, such as albuterol (Ventolin®) and salmeterol (Serevent), relieve bronchospasm and airway obstruction.
- Corticosteroids, both inhaled (Pulmicort®, Vanceril®) and oral (prednisone) may improve symptoms but are used mostly for associated asthma.
- Oxygen therapy may be long term continuous or used during exertion.
- Bullectomy (for bullous emphysema) to remove bullae (enlarged airspaces that do not ventilate).
- Lung volume reduction surgery may be done if involvement in the lung is limited; however, mortality rates are high.
- Lung transplantation is a definitive high-risk option.
- Pulmonary rehabilitation includes breathing exercises, muscle training, activity pacing, and modification of activities.

Chronic Ventilatory Failure

Chronic ventilatory failure occurs when alveolar ventilation fails to increase in response to increasing levels of carbon dioxide, usually associated with chronic pulmonary diseases, such as asthma and COPD, drug overdoses, or diseases that impair respiratory effort, such as Guillain-Barré and myasthenia gravis. Normally, the ventilatory system is able to maintain PCO_2 and pH levels within narrow limits, even though PO_2 levels may be more variable, but with ventilatory failure, the body is not able to compensate for the resultant hypercapnia and pH falls, resulting in respiratory acidosis. Symptoms include increasing dyspnea with tachypnea, gasping respirations, and use of accessory muscles. Patients may become confused as hypercapnia causes increased intracranial pressure. If pH is <7.2, cardiac arrhythmias, hyperkalemia, and hypotension can occur as pulmonary arteries constrict and the peripheral vascular system dilates. Diagnosis is per symptoms, ABGs consistent with respiratory acidosis (PCO_2 >50 and pH <7.35), pulse oximetry, and chest x-ray. Treatment can include non-invasive PPV (BiPAP), endotracheal mechanical ventilation, corticosteroids, and bronchodilators.

Chronic Asthma

The three primary symptoms of chronic asthma are cough, wheezing, and dyspnea. In cough-variant asthma, a severe cough may be the only symptom, at least initially. Chronic asthma is characterized by recurring bronchospasm and inflammation of the airways resulting in airway obstruction. Asthma affects the bronchi and not the alveoli. While no longer considered part of COPD because airway obstruction is not constant and is responsive to treatment, over time fibrotic changes in the airways can result in permanent obstruction, especially if asthma is not treated adequately. **Symptoms** of chronic asthma include nighttime coughing, exertional dyspnea, tightness in the chest, and cough. Acute exacerbations may occur, sometimes related to triggers, such as allergies, resulting in increased dyspnea, wheezing, cough, tachycardia, bronchospasm, and rhonchi. **Treatment** of chronic asthma includes chest hygiene, identification and avoidance of triggers, prompt treatment of infections, bronchodilators, long-acting β-2 agonists, and inhaled glucocorticoids.

Status Asthmaticus

Pathophysiology

Status asthmaticus is a severe acute attack of asthma that does not respond to conventional therapy. An acute attack of asthma is precipitated by some stimulus, such as an antigen that triggers an allergic response, resulting in an inflammatory cascade that causes edema of the mucous membranes (swollen airway), contraction of smooth muscles (bronchospasm), increased mucus production (cough and obstruction), and hyperinflation of airways (decreased ventilation and shunting). Mast cells and T lymphocytes produce cytokines, which continue the inflammatory response through increased blood flow coupled with vasoconstriction and bronchoconstriction, resulting in fluid leakage from the vasculature. Epithelial cells and cilia are destroyed, exposing nerves and causing hypersensitivity. Sympathetic nervous system receptors in the bronchi stimulate bronchodilation.

Clinical Symptoms

The person with status asthmaticus will often present in acute distress, non-responsive to inhaled bronchodilators. **Symptoms** include:

- Signs of airway obstruction
- Sternal and intercostal retractions
- Tachypnea and dyspnea with increasing cyanosis

- Forced prolonged expirations
- Cardiac decompensation with increased left ventricular afterload and increased pulmonary edema resulting from alveolar-capillary permeability. Hypoxia may trigger an increase in pulmonary vascular resistance with increased right ventricular afterload.
- Pulsus paradoxus (decreased pulse on inspiration and increased on expiration) with extra beats on inspiration detected through auscultation but not detected radially. Blood pressure normally decreases slightly during inspiration, but this response is exaggerated. Pulsus paradoxus indicates increasing severity of asthma.
- Hypoxemia (with impending respiratory failure)
- Hypocapnia followed by hypercapnia (with impending respiratory failure)
- Metabolic acidosis

INDICATIONS FOR MECHANICAL VENTILATION FOR STATUS ASTHMATICUS

Mechanical ventilation (MV) for status asthmaticus should be avoided, if possible, because of the danger of increased bronchospasm as well as barotrauma and decreased circulation. However, there are some absolute indications for the use of intubation and ventilation and a number of other indications that are evaluated on an individual basis.

The following are **absolute indications for MV:**

- Cardiac and/or pulmonary arrest
- Markedly depressed mental status (obtundation)
- Severe hypoxia and/or apnea

The following are **relative indications for MV:**

- Exhaustion/muscle fatigue from exertion of breathing
- Sharply diminished breath sounds and no audible wheezing
- Pulse paradoxus >20-40 mmHg; absent = imminent respiratory arrest
- PaO_2 <70 mmHg on 100% oxygen
- Dysphonia
- Central cyanosis
- Increased hypercapnia
- Metabolic/respiratory acidosis: pH <7.20

In this patient population, ventilator goal is to minimize airway pressures while oxygenating the patient. Vent settings include: low tidal volume (6-8 mL/kg), low respiratory rate (10-14 respirations/minute), and high inspiratory flow rate (80-100 L/min).

AIR LEAK SYNDROMES

Air leak syndromes may result in significant respiratory distress. Leaks may occur spontaneously or secondary to some type of trauma (accidental, mechanical, iatrogenic) or disease. As pressure increases inside the alveoli, the alveolar wall pulls away from the perivascular sheath and subsequent alveolar rupture allows air to follow the perivascular planes and flow into adjacent areas. There are two categories:

- **Pneumothorax:**
    - Air in the pleural space causes a lung to collapse.
- **Barotrauma/volutrauma** with air in the interstitial space (usually resolve over time):

- Pneumoperitoneum is air in the peritoneal area, including the abdomen and occasionally the scrotal sac of male infants.
- Pneumomediastinum is air in the mediastinal area between the lungs.
- Pneumopericardium is air in the pericardial sac that surrounds the heart.
- Subcutaneous emphysema is air in the subcutaneous tissue planes of the chest wall.
- Pulmonary interstitial emphysema (PIE) is air trapped in the interstitium between the alveoli.

PNEUMOTHORAX

Pneumothorax occurs when there is a leak of air into the pleural space, resulting in complete or partial collapse of a lung.

Symptoms: Vary widely depending on the cause and degree of the pneumothorax and whether or not there is an underlying disease. Symptoms include acute pleuritic pain (95%), usually on the affected side, and decreased breath sounds. In a *tension pneumothorax,* symptoms include tracheal deviation and hemodynamic compromise.

Diagnosis: Clinical findings; radiograph: 6-foot upright posterior-anterior; ultrasound may detect traumatic pneumothorax.

Treatment: Chest-tube thoracostomy with underwater seal drainage is the most common treatment for all types of pneumothorax.

- Tension pneumothorax: Immediate needle decompression and chest tube thoracostomy
- Small pneumothorax, patient stable: Oxygen administration and observation for 3-6 hours. If no increase is shown on repeat x-ray, patient may be discharged with another x-ray in 24 hours.
- Primary spontaneous pneumothorax: Catheter aspiration or chest tube thoracostomy

PLEURAL EFFUSION AND EMPYEMA

Pleural effusion is the accumulation of fluid in the pleural space, usually secondary to other disease processes, such as heart failure, TB, neoplasms, nephrotic syndrome, and viral respiratory infections. The fluid may be serous, bloody, or purulent (empyema) and transudative or exudative. Signs and symptoms depend on underlying condition but includes dyspnea, from mild to severe. Tracheal deviation away from affected side may be evident. Diagnosis includes chest x-ray, lateral decubitus x-ray, CT, thoracentesis, and pleural biopsy. Treatment includes treating underlying cause, thoracentesis to remove fluid, insertion of chest tube, pleurodesis, or pleurectomy or pleuroperitoneal shunt (primarily with malignancy).

> **Review Video: Pleural Effusions**
> Visit mometrix.com/academy and enter code: 145719

Empyema is a pleural effusion in which the collection of pleural fluid is thick and purulent, usually as a result of bacterial pneumonia or penetrating chest trauma. Empyema may also occur as a complication of thoracentesis or thoracic surgery. Signs and symptoms include acute illness with fever, chills, pain, cough, and dyspnea. Diagnosis is per chest CT and thoracentesis with culture and sensitivity. Treatment includes antibiotics and drainage of pleural space per needle aspiration, tube thoracostomy, or open chest drainage with thoracotomy.

Pulmonary Fibrosis

Pulmonary fibrosis is a progressive disease of the lungs in which scarring of the tissue causes the lining of the lungs to thicken. This thickening prevents adequate oxygen exchange from occurring. The cause of pulmonary fibrosis is unknown, however environmental toxins such as asbestos, infections, smoking and occupational exposure to wood or metal dust may be contributing factors. The disease is more prevalent in males and the average age at the time of diagnosis is between 40 and 70. There may also be a genetic predisposition in the development of pulmonary fibrosis. The median survival for patients diagnosed with pulmonary fibrosis is less than five years.

Signs and symptoms: Shortness of breath, dry cough, fatigue, weight loss, and clubbing of the finger tips and nails.

Diagnosis: Physical assessment, chest x-ray and/or computed tomography, pulmonary function tests, arterial blood gases and lung biopsy.

Treatment: There is no cure for pulmonary fibrosis and treatment options are minimal. Anti-inflammatory medications such as corticosteroids may be used for symptom management as well as supplemental oxygen therapy. Lung transplantation may be an option for some patients based on age and advancement of disease. Some patients may be eligible for participation in a clinical trial, as there are research efforts focused on treatment options to halt the progression of the disease.

Pulmonary Hypertension and Pulmonary Arterial Hypertension

Pulmonary arterial hypertension (PAH) is a progressive disease of the pulmonary arteries that can severely compromise cardiovascular patients. It may involve multiple processes. Usually, the pulmonary vasculature adjusts easily to accommodate blood volume from the right ventricle. If there is increased blood flow, the low resistance causes vasodilation and vice versa. However, sometimes the pulmonary vascular bed is damaged or obstructed, and this can impair the ability to handle changing volumes of blood. In that case, an increase in flow will increase the pulmonary arterial pressure, increasing pulmonary vascular resistance (PVR). This in turn, increases pressure on the right ventricle (RV) with increased RV workload and eventually causes RV hypertrophy with displacement of the intraventricular septum and tricuspid regurgitation (cor pulmonale). Over time, this leads to right heart failure and death. Pulmonary hypertension is usually diagnosed by right-sided heart catheterization and is indicated by systolic pulmonary artery pressure >30 mmHg and mean pulmonary artery pressure >25 mmHg. Non-invasive testing may include echocardiogram to look for cardiac changes.

Types

Pulmonary hypertension or pulmonary arterial hypertension (PAH) may be classified as primary (idiopathic) or secondary.

- **Primary (idiopathic) PAH** may result from changes in immune responses, pulmonary emboli, sickle cell disease, collagen diseases, Raynaud's, and the use of contraceptives. The cause may be unknown or genetic.

- **Secondary PAH** may result from pulmonary vasoconstriction brought on by hypoxemia related to COPD, sleep-disordered breathing, kyphoscoliosis, obesity, smoke inhalation, altitude sickness, interstitial pneumonia, and neuromuscular disorders. It may also be caused by a decrease in pulmonary vascular bed of 50-75%, which may result from pulmonary emboli, vasculitis, tumor emboli, and interstitial lung disease, such as sarcoidosis. Primary cardiac disease, such as congenital defects in infants, and acquired disorders, such as rheumatic valve disease, mitral stenosis, and left ventricular failure may also contribute to PAH.

TREATMENT OPTIONS FOR PAH

Medical treatment for pulmonary arterial hypertension (PAH) aims to identify and treat any underlying cardiac or pulmonary disease, control symptoms, and prevent complications:

- **Oxygen therapy** may be needed, especially supplemental oxygen during exercise.
- **Calcium channel blockers** may provide vasodilation for some patients.
- **Pulmonary vascular dilators**, such as IV epoprostenol (Flolan®) and subcutaneous treprostinil sodium (Remodulin®) and oral bosentan (Tracleer®) help to control symptoms and prolong life.
- **Anticoagulants**, such as warfarin (Coumadin®) are an important part of therapy because of recurrent pulmonary emboli. Studies have shown that anticoagulation increases survival rates.
- **Diuretics**, such as furosemide (Lasix®) may be needed to relieve edema and restrict fluids, especially with right ventricular hypertrophy.

In some patients who cannot be managed adequately through medical treatment, a heart-lung transplant may be considered as the only effective treatment for long-term survival.

Respiratory Procedures and Interventions

NON-INVASIVE VENTILATION
NASAL CANNULA

A nasal cannula can be used to deliver supplemental oxygen to a patient, but it is only useful for flow rates ≤6 L/min as higher rates are drying of the nasal passages. As it is not an airtight system, some ambient air is breathed in as well so oxygen concentration ranges from about 24-44%. The nasal cannula does not allow for control of respiratory rate, so the patient must be able to breathe independently.

NON-REBREATHER MASK

A non-rebreather mask can be used to deliver higher concentrations (60-90%) of oxygen to those patients who are able to breathe independently. The mask fits over the nose and mouth and is secured by an elastic strap. A 1.5 L reservoir bag is attached and connects to an oxygen source. The bag is inflated to about 1 liter at a rate of 8-15 L/min before the mask is applied as the patient breathes from this reservoir. A one-way exhalation valve prevents most exhaled air from being rebreathed.

NON-INVASIVE POSITIVE PRESSURE VENTILATORS

Non-invasive positive pressure ventilators provide air through a tight-fitting nasal or face mask, usually pressure cycled, avoiding the need for intubation and reducing the danger of hospital-acquired infection and mortality rates. It can be used for acute respiratory failure and pulmonary edema. There are 2 types of non-invasive positive pressure ventilators:

- **CPAP (Continuous positive airway pressure)** provides a steady stream of pressurized air throughout both inspiration and expiration. CPAP improves breathing by decreasing preload for patients with congestive heart failure. It reduces the effort required for breathing by increasing residual volume and improving gas exchange.
- **Bi-PAP (Bi-level positive airway pressure)** provides a steady stream of pressurized air as CPAP but it senses inspiratory effort and increases pressure during inspiration. Bi-PAP pressures for inspiration and expiration can be set independently. Machines can be programmed with a backup rate to ensure a set number of respirations per minute.

NEVER place a patient in wrist restraints while wearing these devices. If the patient vomits, they need to be able to remove the mask to prevent aspiration.

FACE MASK

Ensuring that a face mask (Ambu bag) is the correct fit and type is important for adequate ventilation, oxygenation, and prevention of aspiration. Difficulties in management of face mask ventilation relate to risk factors: >55 years, obesity, beard, edentulous, and history of snoring. In some cases, if dentures are adhered well, they may be left in place during induction. The face mask is applied by lifting the mandible (jaw thrust) to the mask and avoiding pressure on soft tissue. Oral or nasal airways may be used, ensuring that the distal end is at the angle of the mandible. There are a number of steps to prevent mask airway leaks:

- Increasing or decreasing the amount of air to the mask to allow better seal
- Securing the mask with both hands while another person ventilates
- Accommodating a large nose by using the mask upside down
- Utilizing a laryngeal mask airway if excessive beard prevents seal

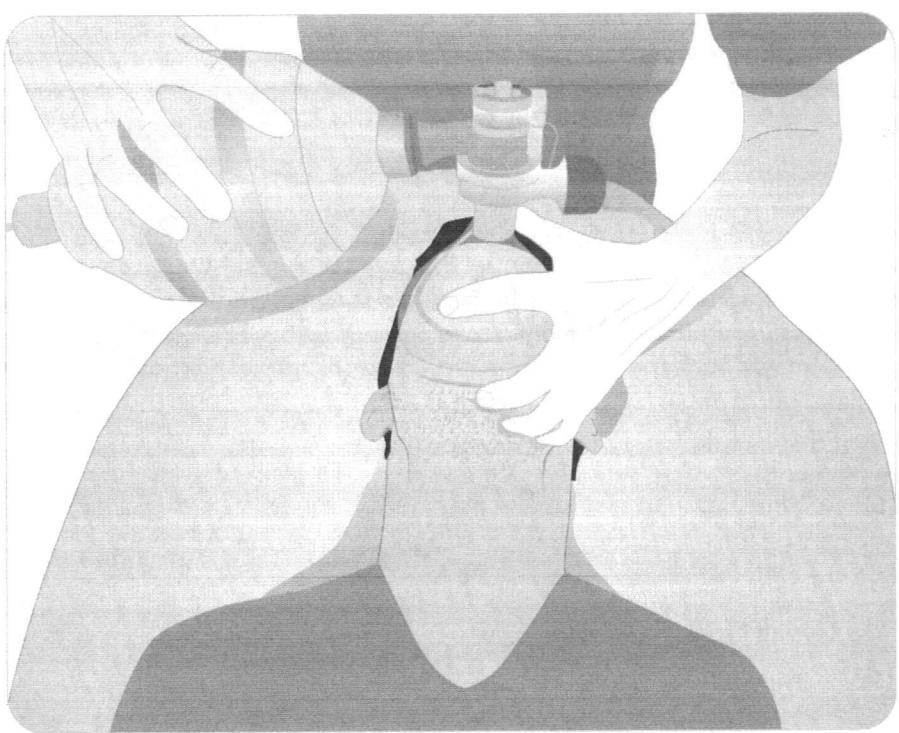

High and Low Flow Oxygen Delivery

High flow oxygen delivery devices provide oxygen at flow rates higher than the patient's inspiratory flow rate at specific medium to high FiO$_2$, up to 100%. However, a flow of 100% oxygen actually provides only 60-80% FiO$_2$ to the patient because the patient also breathes in some room air, diluting the oxygen. The actual amount of oxygen received depends on the type of interface or mask. Additionally, the flow rate is actually less than the inspiratory flow rate upon actual delivery. High flow oxygen delivery is usually not used in the sleep center. Humidification is usually required because the high flow is drying.

Low flow oxygen delivery devices provide 100% oxygen at flow rates lower than the patient's inspiratory flow rate, but the oxygen mixes with room air, so the FiO$_2$ varies. Humidification is usually only required if flow rate is >3L/min. Much oxygen is wasted with exhalation, so a number of different devices to conserve oxygen are available. Interfaces include transtracheal catheters and cannulae with reservoirs.

Airway Devices
Oropharyngeal, Nasopharyngeal, and Tracheostomy Tubes

Airways are used to establish a patent airway and facilitate respirations:

- **Oropharyngeal**: This plastic airway curves over the tongue and creates space between the mouth and the posterior pharynx. It is used for anesthetized or unconscious patients to keep tongue and epiglottis from blocking the airway.
- **Nasopharyngeal** (trumpet): This smaller flexible airway is more commonly used in conscious patients and is inserted through one nostril, extending to the nasopharynx. It is commonly utilized in patients who need frequent suctioning.
- **Tracheostomy tubes**: Tracheostomy may be utilized for mechanical ventilation. Tubes are inserted into the opening in the trachea to provide a conduit and maintain the opening. The tube is secured with ties around the neck. Because the air entering the lungs through the tracheostomy bypasses the warming and moistening effects of the upper airway, air is humidified through a room humidifier or through the delivery of humidified air through a special mask or mechanical ventilation. If the tracheostomy is going to be long-term, eventually a stoma will form at the site, and the tube can be removed.

Laryngeal Mask Airway

The laryngeal-mask airway (LMA) is an intermediate airway allowing ventilation but not complete respiratory control. The LMA consists of an inflatable cuff (the mask) with a connecting tube. It may be used temporarily before tracheal intubation or when tracheal intubation can't be done. It can also be a conduit for later blind insertion of an endotracheal tube. The head and neck must be in neutral position for insertion of the LMA. If the patient has a gag reflex, conscious sedation or topical anesthesia (deep oropharyngeal) is required. The LMA is inserted by sliding along the hard palate, using the finger as a guide, into the pharynx, and the ring is inflated to create a seal about the opening to the larynx, allowing ventilation with mild positive-pressure. The ProSeal® LMA has a modified cuff that extends onto the back of the mask to improve seal. LMA is contraindicated in morbid obesity, obstructions or abnormalities of oropharynx, and non-fasting patients, as some aspiration is possible even with the cuff seal inflated.

Esophageal-Tracheal Combitube®

The esophageal tracheal Combitube® (ETC) is an intermediate airway that contains two lumens and can be inserted into either the trachea or the esophagus (≤91%). The twin-lumen tube has a proximal cuff providing a seal of the oropharynx and a distal cuff providing a seal about the distal tube. Prior to insertion, the Combitube® cuffs should be checked for leaks (15 mL of air into distal and 85 mL of air into proximal). The patient should be non-responsive and with absent gag reflex with head in neutral position. The tube is passed along the tongue and into the pharynx, utilizing markings on the tube (black guidelines) to determine depth by aligning the ETC with the upper incisors or alveolar ridge. Once in place the distal cuff is inflated (10-15 mL) and then placement in the trachea or esophagus should be determined, so the proper lumen for ventilation can be used. The proximal cuff is inflated (usually to 50-75 mL) and ventilation begun. A capnogram should be used to confirm ventilation.

ENDOTRACHEAL INTUBATION

Endotracheal intubation is often necessary with respiratory failure for control of hypoxemia, hypercapnia, hypoventilation, and/or obstructed airway. Equipment should be assembled and tubes and connections checked for air leaks with a 10 mL syringe. The mouth and/or nose should be cleaned of secretions and suctioned if necessary. The patient should be supine with the patient's head level with the lower sternum of the clinician. With orotracheal/endotracheal intubation, the clinician holds the laryngoscope (in left hand) and inserts it into right corner of mouth, the epiglottis is lifted and the larynx exposed. A thin flexible intubation stylet may be used and the endotracheal tube (ETT) (in right hand) is inserted through the vocal cords and into the trachea, cuff inflated to minimal air leak (10 mL initially until patient stabilizes), and placement confirmed through capnometry or esophageal detection devices. The correct depth of insertion is verified: 21 cm (female), 23 cm (male). After insertion, the tube is secured.

> **Review Video: Mechanical Ventilation**
> Visit mometrix.com/academy and enter code: 679637

THORACENTESIS

A thoracentesis (aspiration of fluid or air from pleural space) is done to make a diagnosis, relieve pressure on the lung caused by pleural effusion, or instill medications. A chest x-ray is done prior to the procedure. A sedative may be given. The patient is in a sitting position, leaning onto a padded bedside stand, straddling a chair with head supported on the back of the chair, or lying on the opposite side with the head of the bed elevated 30-45° to ensure that fluid remains at the base. The patient should avoid coughing or moving during the procedure. The chest x-ray or ultrasound determines needle placement. After a local anesthetic is administered, a needle (with an attached 20-mL syringe and 3-way stopcock with tubing and a receptacle) is advanced intercostally into the pleural space. Fluid is drained, collected, examined, and measured. The needle is removed and a pressure dressing applied. A chest x-ray is done to ensure there is no pneumothorax. The patient is monitored for cough, dyspnea, and hypoxemia.

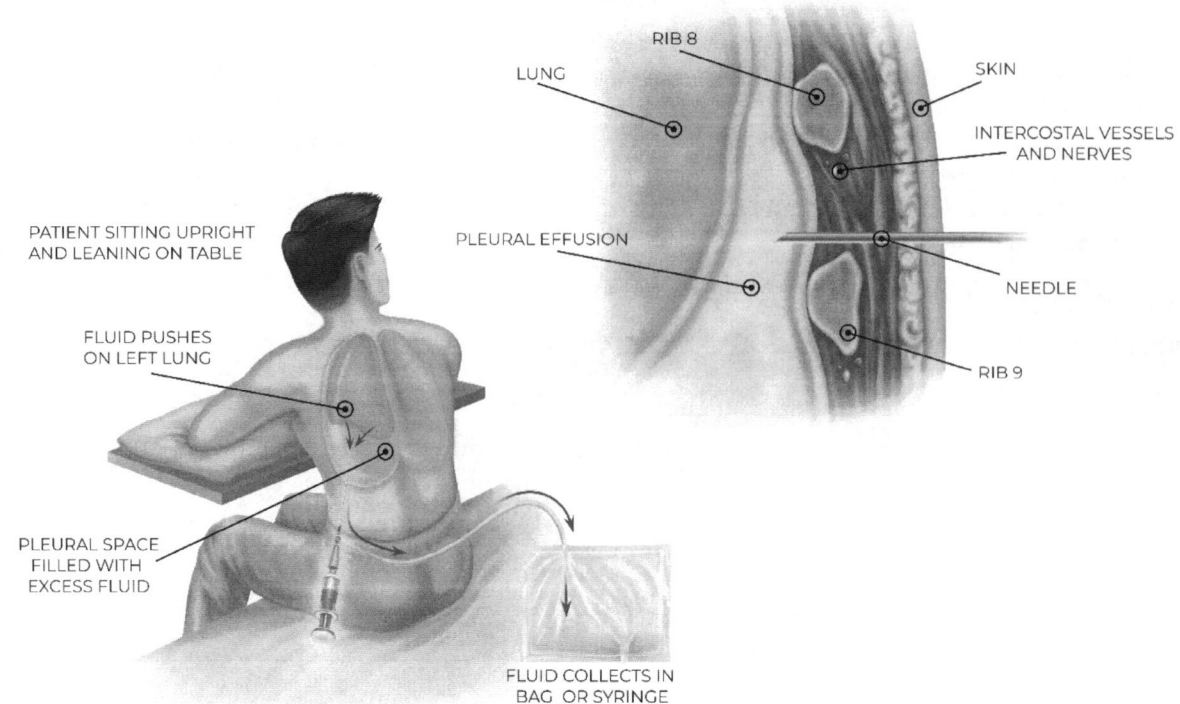

BRONCHOSCOPY

Bronchoscopy utilizes a thin, flexible fiberoptic bronchoscope to inspect the larynx, trachea, and bronchi for diagnostic purposes. It is also used to collect specimens, obtain biopsies, remove foreign bodies or secretions, treat atelectasis, and to excise lesions. The patient is in supine position during the procedure. The Mallampati classification may be used to determine difficulty of airway. The patient receives local anesthesia to the nares (lidocaine gel) and oropharynx (lidocaine gel, spray, or nebulizer), and usually receives a benzodiazepine (commonly midazolam or lorazepam), an opioid (fentanyl or meperidine), or propofol. Medications are usually given in small incremental doses throughout the procedure and may be combined. Over-sedation may cause physiologic depression, but undersedation may result in recall and agitation with sympathetic activation. The tube is advanced through the nares and down the trachea to the bronchi. Airway patency, respiratory rate, and oxygen saturation must be constantly monitored. Complications can include bleeding, arrhythmias, obstruction, laryngospasm, and respiratory failure.

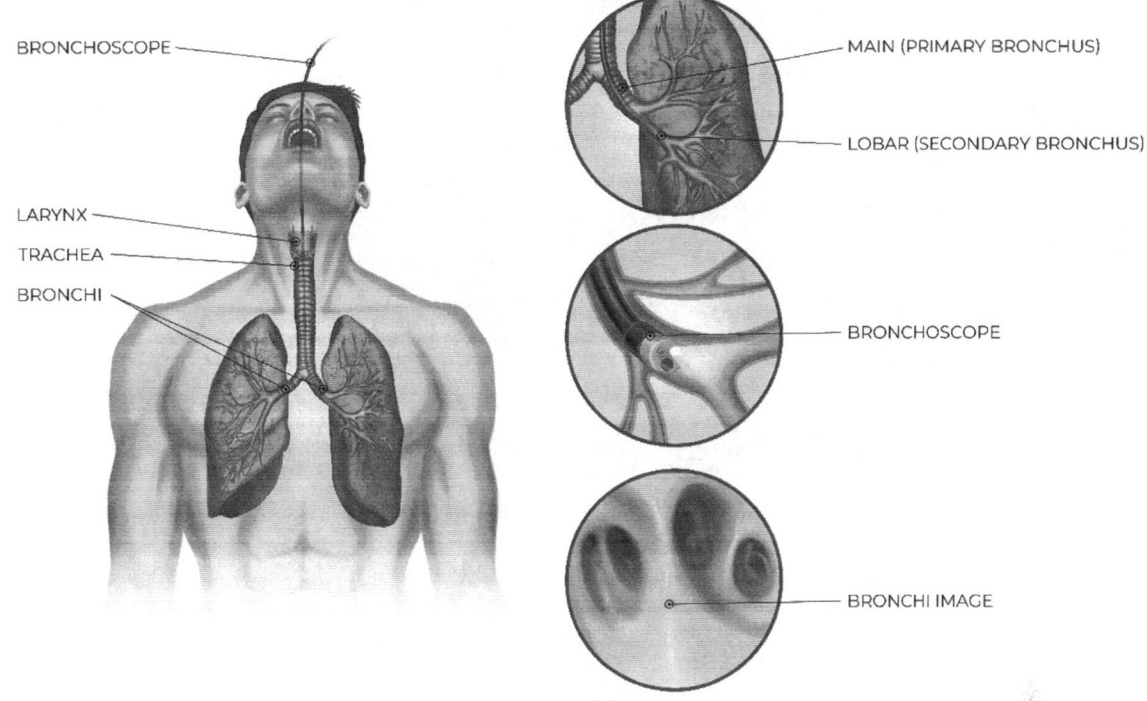

Hematologic Pathophysiology

ANEMIA

Anemia occurs when there is an insufficient number of red blood cells to sufficiently oxygenate the body. As a result of the decreased level of oxygen being supplied to the organs, the body will attempt to compensate by increasing cardiac output and redistributing blood to the brain and heart. In return, the blood supply to the skin, abdominal organs, and kidneys is decreased. Anemia can occur from blood loss, increased destruction of red blood cells (hemolytic anemia), or as a result of a decreased production in red blood cells.

Signs and symptoms: Pallor, fatigue, hypotension, weakness and mental status changes. As perfusion decreases and the body attempts to compensate for the lack of oxygenation, tachycardia, chest pain, and shortness of breath may occur. In hemolytic anemias, jaundice and splenomegaly may occur as the result of the breakdown of red blood cells and the excretion of bilirubin.

Diagnosis: A complete blood count, reticulocyte count, and iron studies may be used to diagnose anemia.

Treatment: The treatment of anemia is focused on treating the underlying cause. Parenteral iron may be given for patients with iron deficiency anemias caused from chronic blood loss, or inadequate iron intake or absorption. Blood transfusions are used to treat patients with active bleeding as well as those patients who are displaying significant clinical symptoms. Erythropoietin stimulating proteins may also be utilized to decrease the need for a transfusion.

SICKLE CELL DISEASE

Sickle cell disease is a recessive genetic disorder of chromosome 11, causing hemoglobin to be defective so that red blood cells (RBCs) are sickle-shaped and inflexible, resulting in their accumulating in small vessels and causing painful blockage. While normal RBCs survive 120 days, sickled cells may survive only 10-20 days, stressing the bone marrow that cannot produce fast enough and resulting in severe anemia. There are 5 variations of sickle cell disease, with sickle cell anemia the most severe. Different types of crises occur (aplastic, hemolytic, vaso-occlusive, and sequestrating), which can cause infarctions in organs, severe pain, damage to organs, and rapid enlargement of liver and spleen. Complications include anemia, acute chest syndrome, congestive heart failure, strokes, delayed growth, infections, pulmonary hypertension, liver and kidney disorders, retinopathy, seizures, and osteonecrosis. Sickle cell disease occurs almost exclusively in African Americans in the United States, with 8-10% carriers.

> **Review Video: Sickle Cell Disease**
> Visit mometrix.com/academy and enter code: 603869

TREATMENT

Treatment for sickle cell disease includes:

- **Prophylactic penicillin** for children from 2 months to 5 years to prevent pneumonia
- **IV fluids** to prevent dehydration
- **Analgesics** (morphine) during painful crises
- **Folic acid** for anemia
- **Oxygen** for congestive heart failure or pulmonary disease
- **Blood transfusions** with chelation therapy to remove excess iron OR erythropheresis, in which red cells are removed and replaced with healthy cells, either autologous or from a donor
- **Hematopoietic stem cells transplantation** is the only curative treatment, but immunosuppressive drugs must be used and success rates are only about 85%, so the procedure is only used on those at high risk. It requires ablation of bone marrow, placing the patient at increased risk.
- **Partial chimerism** uses a mixture of the donor and the recipient's bone marrow stem cells and does not require ablation of bone marrow. It is showing good success.

POLYCYTHEMIA VERA

Polycythemia vera is a condition in which there is abnormal production of blood cells in the bone marrow. Erythrocytes (red blood cells) are primarily affected. The disease is more common in men older than 40 years. Polycythemia may be primary or secondary, related to conditions causing hypoxia. The blood increases in viscosity, resulting in a number of **symptoms**:

- Dizziness, headache, weakness, and fatigue
- Dyspnea, especially when supine
- Flushing of skin, blue-tinged skin discoloration, and red lesions
- Itching after warm bath
- Left upper abdominal fullness and splenomegaly
- Phlebitis from blood clots
- Vision disturbances
- Complications include stroke, hemorrhage, and heart failure

Diagnosis includes CBC with differential, chemistry panel, bone marrow biopsy, and Vitamin B_{12} level. Red cell mass will be more than 25% above normal.

Treatment includes:

- **Phlebotomy** to remove 500 mL (lesser amounts for children) of blood to decrease blood viscosity, repeated weekly until hematocrit stable (less than 45%)
- Referral for **chemotherapy** (hydroxyurea) to suppress marrow production
- **Interferon** to decrease need for phlebotomy

VON WILLEBRAND DISEASE

Von Willebrand disease is a group of congenital bleeding disorders (inherited from either parent) affecting 1-2% of the population, associated with deficiency or lack of von Willebrand factor (vWF), a glycoprotein that is synthesized, stored, and secreted by vascular endothelial cells. This protein interacts with thrombocytes to create a clot and prevent hemorrhage; however, with von Willebrand disease, this clotting mechanism is impaired. There are three types:

- **Type I**: Low levels of vWF and also sometimes factor VIII (dominant inheritance)
- **Type II**: Abnormal vWF (subtypes a, b) may increase or decrease clotting (dominant inheritance)
- **Type III**: Absence of vWF and less than 10% factor VIII (recessive inheritance)

Symptoms vary in severity and include bruising, menorrhagia, recurrent epistaxis, and hemorrhage.

Treatment includes:

- **Desmopressin acetate** parenterally or nasally to stimulate production of clotting factor (mild cases)
- **Severe bleeding**: factor VIII concentrates with vWF, such as Humate-P

HEMOPHILIA

Hemophilia is an inherited disorder in which the person lacks adequate clotting factors. There are three types:

- **Type A**: lack of clotting factor VIII (90% of cases)
- **Type B**: lack of clotting factor IX
- **Type C**: lack of clotting factor XI (affects both sexes, rarely occurs in the United States)

Both Type A and B are usually X-linked disorders, affecting only males. The severity of the disease depends on the amount of clotting factor in the blood.

Symptoms:

- Bleeding with severe trauma or stress (mild cases)
- Unexplained bruises, bleeding, swelling, joint pain
- Spontaneous hemorrhage (severe cases), often in the joints but can be anywhere in the body
- Epistaxis, mucosal bleeding
- First symptoms often occur during infancy when the child becomes active, resulting in frequent bruises

Treatment:

- Desmopressin acetate parenterally or nasally to stimulate production of clotting factor (mild cases)
- Infusions of clotting factor from donated blood or recombinant clotting factors (genetically engineered), utilizing guidelines for dosing
- Infusions of plasma (Type C)

DISSEMINATED INTRAVASCULAR COAGULATION
PATHOLOGY

Disseminated intravascular coagulation (DIC) (consumption coagulopathy) is a secondary disorder that is triggered by another disorder such as trauma, congenital heart disease, necrotizing enterocolitis, sepsis, and severe viral infections. DIC triggers both coagulation and hemorrhage through a complex series of events. Trauma causes tissue factor (transmembrane glycoprotein) to enter the circulation and bind with coagulation factors, triggering the coagulation cascade. This stimulates thrombin to convert fibrinogen to fibrin, causing aggregation and destruction of platelets and forming clots that can be disseminated throughout the intravascular system. These clots increase in size as platelets adhere to the clots, causing blockage of both the microvascular systems and larger vessels, which can result in ischemia and necrosis. Clot formation triggers fibrinolysis and plasmin to breakdown fibrin and fibrinogen, causing the destruction of clotting factors and resulting in hemorrhage. Both processes, clotting and hemorrhage, continue at the same time, placing the patient at high risk for death, even with treatment.

SYMPTOMS AND TREATMENT

The onset of symptoms of DIC may be very rapid or be a slower chronic progression from a disease. Those who develop the chronic manifestation of the disease usually have fewer acute symptoms and may slowly develop ecchymosis or bleeding wounds.

Symptoms include:

- Bleeding from surgical or venous puncture sites
- Evidence of GI bleeding with distention, bloody diarrhea
- Hypotension and acute symptoms of shock
- Petechiae and purpura with extensive bleeding into the tissues
- Laboratory abnormalities:
    - Prolonged prothrombin and partial prothrombin times
    - Decreased platelet counts and fragmented RBCs
    - Decreased fibrinogen

Treatment includes:

- Identifying and treating underlying cause
- Massive blood transfusion protocol; replacement of blood products, such as platelets and fresh frozen plasma
- Anticoagulation therapy (heparin) to increase clotting time
- Cryoprecipitate to increase fibrinogen levels
- Coagulation inhibitors and coagulation factors

Thrombocytopenia

Thrombocytopenia is a deficiency of circulating platelets in the blood. It can be caused by a decrease in the production of platelets from the bone marrow or an increase in destruction of platelets. Thrombocytopenia may also be caused from the use of heparin. Heparin induced thrombocytopenia can occur after heparin therapy (average 4-14 days post therapy) and is characterized by a decrease in platelet count to less than 50% of baseline or the occurrence of an unexplained thrombolytic event. A decreased production of platelets within the bone marrow can occur as a result of malignancy, bone marrow failure, infection, alcohol abuse, or a nutritional deficiency. An increase in the destruction of platelets may occur in disseminated intravascular coagulation, vasculitis, thrombotic thrombocytopenic purpura, sepsis, or idiopathic thrombocytopenic purpura.

Signs and symptoms: Signs and symptoms may include petechiae, ecchymosis, bleeding from the mouth or gums, epistaxis, pallor, weakness, fatigue, splenomegaly, blood in the urine or stool, and jaundice.

Diagnosis: Physical exam and lab studies including complete blood count, partial thromboplastin time and prothrombin time may be used to diagnosis thrombocytopenia. A bone marrow biopsy may be indicated to determine the cause of the decreased production of platelets.

Treatment: Treatment of thrombocytopenia involves identifying and treating the underlying cause. Medications that decrease the platelet count should be held. Platelet transfusions may be administered to patients with extremely low counts (less than 50,000) or if spontaneous bleeding occurs. Platelet transfusions are contraindicated in patients with thrombotic thrombocytopenia purpura.

ITP

The autoimmune disorder **idiopathic thrombocytopenic purpura (ITP)** causes an immune response to platelets, resulting in decreased platelet counts. ITP affects primarily children and young women although it can occur at any age. The acute form primarily occurs in children, but the chronic form affects primarily adults. Platelet counts are usually 150,000–400,000 per mcL. With ITP, platelet levels are less than 100,000. Maintaining a platelet count of at least 30,000 is necessary to prevent intracranial hemorrhage, the primary concern. The cause of ITP is unclear and may be precipitated by viral infection, sulfa drugs, and conditions, such as lupus erythematosus. ITP is usually not life threatening and can be controlled. **Symptoms** include:

- Bruising and petechiae with hematoma in some cases
- Epistaxis
- Increased menstrual flow in post-puberty females

Treatment includes:

- Corticosteroids to depress immune response and increase platelet count
- Splenectomy may be indicated for chronic conditions
- Platelet transfusions
- Avoiding aspirin, ibuprofen, or other NSAIDs

HITTS

Heparin-induced thrombocytopenia and thrombosis syndrome (HITTS) occurs in patients receiving heparin for anticoagulation. There are two types:

- **Type I** is a transient condition occurring within a few days and causing depletion of platelets (<100,000 mm^3), but heparin may be continued as the condition usually resolves without intervention.
- **Type II** is an autoimmune reaction to heparin that occurs in 3–5% of those receiving unfractionated heparin and also occurs with low-molecular-weight heparin. It is characterized by low platelets (<50,000 mm^3) that are ≥50% below baseline. Onset is 5–14 days but can occur within hours of heparinization. Death rates are <30%. Heparin-antibody complexes form and release platelet factor 4 (PF4), which attracts heparin molecules and adheres to platelets and endothelial lining, stimulating thrombin and platelet clumping. This puts the patient at risk for thrombosis and vessel occlusion rather than hemorrhage, causing stroke, myocardial infarction, and limb ischemia with symptoms associated with the site of thrombosis. Treatment includes:
    - Discontinuation of heparin
    - Direct thrombin inhibitors (lepirudin, argatroban)
    - Monitor for signs/symptoms of thrombus/embolus

REOPRO-INDUCED COAGULOPATHY

ReoPro® (abciximab) is used to prevent cardiac ischemia for those undergoing percutaneous cardiac intervention by inhibiting the aggregation of platelets. It is used with aspirin and/or weight-adjusted low dose heparin and potentiates the action of anticoagulants. However, its use with non-weight adjusted, longer acting heparin can cause thrombocytopenia with increased risk of hemorrhage, especially with readministration of the drug, which can induce the formation of antibodies and an allergic reaction that is characterized by anaphylaxis and thrombocytopenia, referred to as **ReoPro-induced coagulopathy**. Because of the danger of hemorrhage, ReoPro® is contraindicated if there is active bleeding or a history of bleeding or CVA within the 2 years prior, history of a CVA, platelet count <100,000 mm^3, or recent history of oral anticoagulation. Careful monitoring of platelet counts prior to administration and the use of weight-adjusted low dose heparin is important to prevent bleeding. Heparin should be discontinued after the PCI.

Hematologic Procedures and Interventions

TRANSFUSION COMPONENTS

Blood components that are commonly used for transfusions include:

- **Packed red blood cells:** RBCs (250-300 mL per unit) should be warmed >30 °C (optimal 37 °C) before administration to prevent hypothermia and may be reconstituted in 50-100 mL of normal saline to facilitate administration. RBCs are necessary if blood loss is about 30% (1,500-2,000 mL lost; Hgb ≤7). Above 30% blood loss, whole blood may be more effective. RBCs are most frequently used for transfusions.

- **Platelet concentrates:** Transfusions of platelets are used if the platelet count is <50,000 cells/mm³. One unit increases the platelet count by 5,000-10,000 cells/mm³. Platelet concentrates pose a risk for sensitization reactions and infectious diseases. Platelet concentrate is stored at a higher temperature (20-24 °C) than RBCs. This contributes to bacterial growth, so it is more prone to bacterial contamination than other blood products and may cause sepsis. Temperature increase within 6 hours should be considered an indication of possible sepsis. ABO compatibility should be observed but is not required.
- **Fresh frozen plasma** (FFP) (obtained from a unit of whole blood frozen ≤6 hours after collection) includes all clotting factors and plasma proteins, so each unit administered increases clotting factors by 2-3%. FFP may be used for deficiencies of isolated factors, excess warfarin therapy, and liver-disease-related coagulopathy. It may be used for patients who have received extensive blood transfusions but continue to hemorrhage. It is also helpful for those with antithrombin III deficiency. FFP should be warmed to 37 °C prior to administration to avoid hypothermia. ABO compatibility should be observed if possible, but it is not required. Some patients may become sensitized to plasma proteins.
- **Cryoprecipitate** is the precipitate that forms when FFP is thawed. It contains fibrinogen, factor VIII, von Willebrand, and factor XIII. This component may be used to treat hemophilia A and hypofibrinogenemia.

Transfusion Administration

Prior to the transfusion of any blood component, the nurse should obtain the patient's transfusion history along with a consent form. A type and crossmatch must be completed on the patient's blood and an IV in place for administration. An 18-gauge catheter is standard, but 22-gauge can also be used at a slower rate. Baseline vital signs need to be taken prior to starting the infusion, and then the patient should be under direct observation for at least the first 15 minutes. Vital signs should be monitored at 5 minutes, 15 minutes, and then at least every 30 minutes during the transfusion and one hour post-transfusion.

Blood Conservation

Blood conservation includes methods to:

- **Minimize the loss of blood during surgical procedures:** May include regional anesthesia instead of general, positioning to reduce blood loss, cell salvage, autotransfusion, non-invasive monitoring (BP, pulse oximetry), limited blood draws, normovolemic hemodilution, and medications to reduce bleeding (vitamin K, tranexamic acid, desmopressin, somatostatin, vasopressin, recombinant factor VIIa).
- **Lower the threshold for receiving transfusions:** Transfusion threshold lowered from 10 to 7 g/dL.
- **Maintain the hematocrit at acceptable levels:** Administration of oral or parenteral iron therapy to increase tolerance for blood loss. Erythropoietin alpha may also be administered perioperatively to stimulate the production of RBCs.
- **Ensure optimal oxygenation of tissue:** Hyperoxic ventilation during surgery, crystalloid/colloid volume replacement, and utilizing techniques to minimize consumption of oxygen.

Blood conservation includes a commitment to bloodless surgery as much as possible, especially through the utilization of minimally-invasive procedures.

TRANSFUSION-RELATED COMPLICATIONS

There are a number of transfusion-related complications, which is the reason that transfusions are given only when necessary. Complications include:

- **Infection**: Bacterial contamination of blood, especially platelets, can result in severe sepsis. A number of infective agents (viral, bacterial, and parasitic) can be transmitted, although increased testing of blood has decreased rates of infection markedly. Infective agents include HIV, hepatitis C and B, human T-cell lymphotropic virus, CMV, WNV, malaria, Chagas' disease, and variant Creutzfeldt-Jacob disease (from contact with mad cow disease).
- **Transfusion-related acute lung injury (TRALI)**: This respiratory distress syndrome occurs ≤6 hours after transfusion. The cause is believed to be antileukocytic or anti-HLA antibodies in the transfusion. It is characterized by non-cardiogenic pulmonary edema (high protein level) with severe dyspnea and arterial hypoxemia. Transfusion must be stopped immediately and the blood bank notified. TRALI may result in fatality but usually resolves in 12-48 hours with supportive care.
- **Graft vs. host disease**: Lymphocytes cause an immune response in immunocompromised individuals. Lymphocytes may be inactivated by irradiation, as leukocyte filters are not reliable.
- **Post-transfusion purpura**: Platelet antibodies develop and destroy the patient's platelets, so the platelet count decreases about 1 week after transfusion.
- **Transfusion-related immunosuppression**: Cell-mediated immunity is suppressed, so the patient is at increased risk of infection, and in cancer patients, transfusions may correlate with tumor recurrence. This condition relates to transfusions that include leukocytes. RBCs cause a less pronounced immunosuppression, suggesting a causative agent is in the plasma. Leukoreduction is becoming more common to reduce transmission of leukocyte-related viruses.
- **Hypothermia**: This may occur if blood products are not heated. Oxygen utilization is halved for each 10 °C decrease in normal body temperature.

Immunologic and Oncologic Pathophysiology

IMMUNE DEFICIENCIES

There are multiple disorders that fall into the category of **primary immunodeficiency diseases.** These disorders are genetic or inherited disorders in which the body's immune system does not function properly. These disorders may involve low levels of antibodies, defects in the antibodies, or defects in cells that make up the immune system (T-cells, B-cells). Common variable immune deficiency is a common immune deficiency diagnosed in adulthood. This disorder is characterized by low levels of serum immunoglobins and antibodies, which substantially increases the risk of infection.

- **Signs and symptoms**: Recurrent infections are the hallmark sign of immune deficiency disorders. Recurrent infections most often involve the ears, sinuses, bronchi, and lungs. Lymphadenopathy may occur as well as splenomegaly. GI symptoms may include abdominal pain, nausea, vomiting, diarrhea, and weight loss. Some patients may experience polyarthritis. Granulomas are also common and may occur in the lungs, lymph nodes, liver, and skin.

- **Diagnosis**: A physical assessment and patient history are used to diagnose immune deficiency disorders. Since immune deficiency disorders are genetic or inherited, family history should also be evaluated. Lab tests such as serum antibodies, serum immunoglobin levels and a complete blood count may also be used to assist in the diagnosis of immune deficiency disorders.
- **Treatment**: Patients with immune deficiency disorders often receive immunoglobulin replacement. Long term antibiotics may also be administered for recurrent infections. Educate patients to frequently wash hands, cook foods thoroughly, avoid large crowds, and other infection prevention techniques.

CONGENITAL IMMUNODEFICIENCIES

Congenital immunodeficiencies include:

- **Common variable immunodeficiency** is primarily an IgG deficiency due to absent plasma cells and B cell differentiation. These patients have increased susceptibility to encapsulated organisms and are more likely to develop bronchiectasis from the recurrent damage. They are also at higher risk for B cell neoplasms, GI malignancy, and autoimmune disease. Test is with functional antibody response and treatment with IVIG.
- **Congenital Agammaglobulinemia** (Bruton's, x-linked) usually leads to a susceptibility to recurrent pyogenic infections and low IgG and no IgA, IgM, IgE, IgD, or B cells.
- **Selective IgA deficiency** is the most common Ig deficiency and leads to recurrent sinopulmonary infections. It has association with recurrent giardiasis, GI malignancy, and autoimmune disorders, including celiac sprue. One should withhold IVIG due to possible anaphylactic reaction to IgA.
- **Wiskott-Aldrich syndrome** is the combination of thrombocytopenia, eczema, and immunodeficiency. It has associated low IgM and elevated IgA and IgE. BMT treats this successfully.

COMPLEMENT DEFICIENCIES

There are deficiencies of all parts of the complement pathway, including the following:

- **Classical deficiency** may include C1 (q, r, s), C2, and C4. This leads to immune complex syndromes and pyogenic infection, such as recurrent sinopulmonary infections with encapsulated bacteria. There is an association with SLE and other rheumatoid diseases. C2 is the most common deficiency in Caucasians in the US.
- **C3 and alternative complement deficiency** may lead to immune complex syndromes and recurrent infections, such as severe pyogenic infections. It may also be associated with HUS.
- **Membrane attack complex (MAC) deficiency** is also known as terminal complement deficiency. This is associated with recurrent Neisseria infections (which can cause meningitis and sepsis) and immune complex diseases. The CH50 assay must be checked to determine the activity of the classical pathway. CH50 may also be used to follow disease activity in SLE.

AUTOIMMUNE SYSTEM DISORDERS

Allergic interstitial/tubulointerstitial nephritis is inflammation and edema of the interstitial areas of the kidneys. Up to 92% of cases caused by allergic reaction to medications, such as antibiotics (B-lactams, fluoroquinolones, macrolides, and anti-tuberculin drugs), antivirals, NSAIDs, PPIs, antiepileptics, diuretics, chemotherapy, and allopurinol. **Symptoms** include fever, rash, and renal enlargement as well as fatigue, nausea, vomiting, and weight loss. **Diagnosis** is by renal biopsy. Urine tests may show eosinophils, blood, RBC casts and sterile pyuria. Increased protein may be seen in response to NSAIDs. **Treatment** is primarily supportive but requires stopping the triggering medication.

Eosinophilic esophagitis is the accumulation of eosinophils in the esophagus, resulting in chronic inflammation. Damage from proteins produced in esophageal tissue causes scarring and narrowing, resulting in dysphagia, vomiting, choking, GERD, upper abdominal pain, heartburn, and regurgitation. **Causes** include allergic reaction to pollens or foods. **Risk factors** include cold/dry climate, male gender, family history, allergies, and asthma. **Diagnosis** is per endoscopy with biopsy. Blood tests may help confirm allergic reactions. **Treatment** may include dietary limitations, PPIs, and topical steroids. Some may require dilation of the esophagus.

Churg-Strauss syndrome (AKA **eosinophilic granulomatosis with polyangiitis**) is an idiopathic form of pulmonary vasculitis that can affect multiple systems (skin and lungs most often) as well as affecting small- and medium-sized arteries in those with asthma. **Symptoms** include dyspnea, chest pain, skin rash, myopathy, arthropathy, rhinitis, sinusitis, abdominal pain, blood in stools, and paresthesia (from the involvement of nerves). The syndrome is characterized by eosinophilia >1500 cells/mcL or >10% of peripheral total WBC count. X-rays or CTs may show transient opacities or multiple nodules. Tissue biopsies typically show allergic granulomas. **Treatment** usually begins with corticosteroids but other immunosuppressive drugs (cyclophosphamide, methotrexate, azathioprine) may be used, especially if critical organs are involved. The goal of treatment is remission, but patients usually need to take drugs at least 2 years before they are tapered off of the drugs. Up to 50% of patients have relapses.

NEUTROPENIA

Neutropenia is identified as a **polymorphonuclear neutrophil count** equal to or less than 500/mL. **Chronic neutropenia** is a sustained condition of minimal neutrophils lasting 3 or more months. Neutropenia may occur from a decreased production of **white blood cells** (e.g., from chemotherapy or radiation therapy). It may also occur from a loss of white blood cells from autoimmune disease processes. Neutropenia is silent but dangerous. It leaves essentially no neutrophils to fight any threat of infection. Neutrophils make up as much as 70% of the white blood cells circulating in the blood. Neutropenia can be the cause of a septic situation, which can be life-threatening. Up to 70% of patients experiencing a fever while in a neutropenic state will die within 48 hours if not treated aggressively.

LEUKOPENIA

Leukopenia is defined as a decrease in white blood cells. Neutropenia is defined as a low number of neutrophils and is often used interchangeably with the term leukopenia. With a decrease in the number of circulating white blood cells, the patient is at an increased risk for the development of an infection. Leukopenia and neutropenia can occur from either a decrease in the production of white blood cells or an increase in their destruction. Infections, malignancy, autoimmune disorders, medications (including chemotherapy) and a history of radiation therapy may contribute to the development of leukopenia/neutropenia.

Signs and symptoms: Malaise, fever, chills, night sweats, shortness of breath, headache, cough, abdominal pain, tachycardia, and hypotension. A patient with neutropenia/leukopenia is at risk for the development of infections including pneumonia, skin infections, urinary tract infections and gastrointestinal infections. In addition, the patient is at an increased risk for sepsis.

Diagnosis: Complete blood count including an absolute neutrophil count. In addition, a bone marrow biopsy may be performed to determine the cause of the decrease in neutrophils.

Treatment: Supportive therapy is used in the treatment of leukopenia including the aggressive treatment of infections that may develop. Precautions should be taken to protect the patient from additional infections, including strict adherence to sterile technique and infection control procedures. Hematopoietic growth factors may also be given to stimulate the production of neutrophils.

LYMPHEDEMA

Lymphedema results from untreated or incurable **edema**. It is a chronic condition marked by swelling and accumulated fluids within the tissue. This accumulation is a result of lymphatic drainage failure, inadequate lymph transport capacity, an increased lymph production, or a combination of these. Primary disease is a result of **inadequately developed lymphatic pathways**, while the secondary disease process is due to **damage outside of the pathways**. The process is worsened and complicated as **macrophages** are released to control inflammation caused by the increased release of fibroblasts and keratinocytes. There is a gradual increase in adipose tissue and leakage of lymph through the skin. The skin and tissues gradually thicken and change in color, texture, tone, and temperature. It begins to blister and produce hyperkeratosis, warts, papillomatosis, and elephantiasis. There is an ever-increasing risk of infection and further complications.

HIV/AIDS

AIDS is a progression of infection with **human immunodeficiency virus** (HIV). AIDS is diagnosed when the following criteria are met:

- HIV infection
- CD4 count less than 200 cells/mm^3
- AIDS defining condition, such as opportunistic infections (cytomegalovirus, tuberculosis), wasting syndrome, neoplasms (Kaposi sarcoma), or AIDS dementia complex

Because there is such a wide range of AIDS defining conditions, the patient may present with many types of **symptoms**, depending upon the diagnosis, but more than half of AIDS patients exhibit:

- Fever
- Lymphadenopathy
- Pharyngitis
- Rash
- Myalgia/arthralgia
- It is important to review the following:
    - CD4 counts to determine immune status
    - WBC and differential for signs of infection
    - Cultures to help identify any infective agents
    - CBC to evaluate for signs of bleeding or thrombocytopenia

Treatment aims to cure or manage opportunistic conditions and control underlying HIV infection through highly active anti-retroviral therapy (HAART), 3 or more drugs used concurrently.

HODGKIN'S DISEASE

Hodgkin's disease (HD) (lymphoma) is cancer originating in the lymphatic system, resulting in impairment of the immune system. The cancer eventually spreads outside the lymphatic system to other organs. With HD, the lymphatic system produces large abnormal B cells (Reed-Sternberg cells), impairing the ability of the body to produce antibodies. **Diagnosis** may include biopsy of enlarged nodes, CBC, radiographs, CT scan, MRI, gallium scan to show spread of HD, PET scan, and bone marrow biopsy.

Symptoms:

- Painless, enlarged lymph nodes (neck, axillary, clavicular, and femoral areas), sometimes to greater than 1 inch in diameter, with enlargement progressing from one nodal group to another
- Fever with chills and night sweats
- Anorexia
- Pruritus, weakness and fatigue, opportunistic infections
- Other symptoms relate to the area affected by the lymphoma, such as chest pain, cough and dyspnea, or abdominal pain and swelling

Treatment:

- Stabilizing patient
- Treating opportunistic infections
- Referral to oncology/radio-therapy for radiation and chemotherapy

LEUKEMIA

Leukemia is a condition in which the proliferating cells compete with normal cells for nutrition. Leukemia affects all cells because the abnormal cells in the bone marrow depress the formation of all elements, resulting in several consequences, regardless of the type of leukemia:

- Decrease in production of **erythrocytes** (RBCs), resulting in anemia
- Decrease in **neutrophils**, resulting in increased risk of infection
- Decrease in **platelets**, with subsequent decrease in clotting factors and increased bleeding
- Increased risk of **physiological fractures** because of invasion of bone marrow that weakens the periosteum
- Infiltration of **liver, spleen, and lymph glands**, resulting in enlargement and fibrosis
- Infiltration of the **CNS**, resulting in increased intracranial pressure, ventricular dilation, and meningeal irritation with headaches, vomiting, papilledema, nuchal rigidity, and coma progressing to death
- **Hypermetabolism** that deprives cells of nutrients, resulting in anorexia, weight loss, muscle atrophy, and fatigue

> **Review Video: Leukemia**
> Visit mometrix.com/academy and enter code: 940024

RELATIONSHIP OF LEUKOCYTOSIS TO LEUKEMIA

Leukemia occurs when one type of WBC proliferates with immature cells, with the defect occurring in the hematopoietic stem cell, either lymphoid or myeloid. Usually, leukemias classified as blast cell or stem cell refer to lymphoid defects. With acute leukemia, WBC count remains low because the cells are halted at the blast stage and the disease progresses rapidly. Chronic leukemia progresses more slowly and most cells are mature.

Lung Cancer
SCLC
Small cell lung cancer (SCLC) is a rapidly-growing variant of lung cancer found in about 15% of new cases. Its origin is in the bronchi and this type of lung cancer occurs predominantly in smokers. At the time of diagnosis, the disease is usually symptomatic and metastases have generally already occurred. There are 3 subtypes of SCLC: oat cell or small-cell carcinoma, intermediate cell, and small cell combined with squamous cell carcinoma or adenocarcinoma. Differential diagnosis includes tests to distinguish it from slower-growing non-small cell lung cancer, lymphoma, sarcoidosis, metastases due to other primary tumors, or infectious processes. In addition to routine procedures like history, physical examination, and laboratory tests, SCLC is generally staged using imaging tests. In particular, a CT scan with contrast is done to assess the involvement in the lung and other sites, and an MRI of the brain and/or a bone scan may also be done to look for metastases. A bone marrow biopsy may also be indicated.

NSCLC
Non-small cell lung cancer (NSCLC) is a blanket term for several histological types of lung cancer not classified as SCLC. The major histological variants are adenocarcinoma, squamous cell carcinoma, and large cell. The large cell type is anaplastic, which means the cells are relatively undifferentiated. Diagnosis of NSCLCs includes exclusion of small cell lung carcinoma, metastatic lung lesions from other primary sources, sarcoidosis, and infections. The clinician generally stages the disease through use of history, physical examination, and laboratory tests. Imaging studies usually include not only CT scans but also positron emission tomography (PET) and, if metastases are suspected, a brain MRI and possibly a bone scan. Mediastinal node biopsies are generally performed if the PET scan indicates later stage disease; various types of incisions can be made, such as those into the sternum or mediastinum.

Breast Cancer
Staging
The American Joint Committee on Cancer **TNM Staging** has recently developed a complex staging classification for breast cancer. In general, however, early invasive breast cancer would be Stage I or II (IIA or IIB). In these stages, there is either no lymph node involvement or only same-side axillary region lymph node involvement with no distant metastases. Nevertheless, diagnostic tests should include bilateral mammography (and possibly other imaging techniques), blood profiles, hepatic and renal function tests, serum alkaline phosphatase levels, and lymph node biopsy or mapping. Assays for prognostic factors like high levels of HER2 or hormone receptors may also be done. Management is surgery that either conserves the breast or a modified radical mastectomy in which the pectoral muscles are not removed. If there is nodal involvement or other factors exist (such as positive hormone receptors or large tumor size), adjuvant chemotherapy or endocrine treatment is added.

Locally Advanced or Recurrent Breast Cancer or Distant Metastases
Locally advanced stage III breast cancer is a comprehensive term for a highly heterogeneous grouping. All Stage III patients have either some sort of nodal involvement and/or their tumor has extended into the chest wall or skin. They do not have distant metastases. Once the disease has reached this stage, multiple treatment strategies are needed, including chemotherapy (and endocrine therapy in receptor-positive women), surgery, and radiation. Locally recurrent breast cancer, on the other hand, is generally due to insufficient removal of the primary lesion (such as with breast conservation surgery); it can often be managed with further surgery, although other

modalities may be needed if there has been nodal or metastatic spread. Once there is metastatic involvement, therapies are merely palliative and the prognosis is poor.

Prostate Cancer

At present, about one out of nine men will develop **prostate cancer** at some point, and approximately 2-3% of those will die of the disease. There are familial groupings of prostate cancer; for example, mutations in the RNASEL and MSR1 loci coding for host response to infection appear to predispose a man to prostate cancer. Diet affects susceptibility to prostate cancer; in particular, consumption of red meat cooked at high temperature to release aromatic compounds is highly correlated to development of the cancer. Ethnicity may play a role, as African Americans in the U. S. have an especially high rate of prostate cancer, but this may be due in part to diet.

Mechanisms That Contribute to Development of Prostate Cancer

Germline mutations in the RNASEL and MSR1 genes have been associated with an increased risk of developing prostate cancer. There is some evidence that inflammation and infection may play a role in the progression of the disease, and development of lesions termed proliferate inflammatory atrophy (PIA) may predispose a man to later prostate intraepithelial neoplasia and prostate cancer. Molecular changes have also been closely associated with disease progression. These include somatic inactivation of the GSTP1 gene, which fosters susceptibility to oxidant and electron-accepting carcinogens and depression of various functions caused by gene mutations, such as the PTEN tumor-suppressor gene, NKA3.1, and CDKN1B. As discussed previously, screening tests include serum prostate-specific antigen (PSA) levels and digital rectal examination. Diagnosis is generally confirmed by core needle biopsy.

Staging and Grading

There are two **staging systems** that are commonly used for prostate cancer.

- The **TNM system**, which is adapted to many types of cancer, defines the primary tumor (T) when observable as T1 (identified only by histology or needle biopsy), T2 (limited to the prostate), T3 (reaches through the prostate capsule) or T4 (invasion of adjacent structures). The TMN system also expresses regional lymph node involvement from N1 to N3 and distant metastases as M1 if present. An *X* after the T, N, or M indicates inability to assess and a zero means no evidence of presence.
- The **American Urological Association or AUA staging system** classifies prostate cancer in four stages. These stages are fairly similar to the primary tumor staging of the TMN program. Basically, Stage A is disease that is not clinically observable. Stage B is a tumor confined within the prostate gland. Stage C involves malignancy that extends outside the prostate capsule but remains within the area. Stage D is malignancy with metastatic involvement. A Gleason score is a combined measurement of histological grading of the two most prevalent differentiation patterns; a lower score reflects a higher amount of differentiation and each component can be graded from 1 to 5.

Colon Cancer

The factor most closely associated with development of **colon cancer** is age, with about 9 out 10 cases identified after age 50. The vast majority of cases have not been correlated to any heritable gene mutation. However, there is a several-fold increase in risk of development of the disease when a close relative is affected, and there are several familial syndromes related to colon cancer (most notably familial adenomatous polyposis or FAP and HNPCC or hereditary nonpolyposis colon cancer). Risk of colon cancer has been associated with certain dietary practices, including high intake of low fiber and high fat foods. It has also been associated with environmental influences, such as exposure to tobacco. The disease often develops through mutations attributable to either chromosomal instability or to a lesser extent microsatellite (repetitive DNA sequence) instability. The genetic change most often found in patients with both precursor adenomatous polyps or actual colon cancer is a defective APC tumor suppressor locus.

PROCEDURES FOR PREVENTION, DIAGNOSIS, AND STAGING OF COLON CANCER

Identification of individuals with familial syndromes or known genetic changes associated with colon cancer is theoretically a means of preventing colon cancer. Realistically, at present this is rarely done. COX-2 inhibitors, which are basically anti-inflammatory agents, are sometimes used as chemo preventive drugs. Patients usually present with symptoms like anemia, fatigue, weight loss, or changes in bowel habits. A small portion of them have other cancers and up to 40% have polyps in addition to the primary tumor. Colonoscopy is suggested as a diagnostic procedure every 10 years beginning at age 50, and it involves inspection of the entire large intestine using a flexible fiberoptic endoscope. Benign polyps, possible cancer precursors, can be immediately excised. Other diagnostic probes include sigmoidoscopy and virtual colonoscopy. Staging is usually done utilizing imaging techniques like CT scans, MRIs, or PET scans. Liver metastases, common in conjunction with colorectal cancers, can be best visualized using intraoperative ultrasound.

STAGING

There are several classification systems for **staging** colorectal cancers. The most common scheme utilized is the Astler-Coller modified Duke's system. The emphasis of this classification scheme is the depth of tumor invasion into the colon wall. The modified Astler-Coller (MAC), the traditional Duke, and the American Joint Committee on Cancer or AJCC (based on TMN) classification schemes are interrelated. According to Astler-Coller, MAC A is comprised of lesions limited to the mucosa or sub mucosa; MAC B1 and B2 involve extension into or through the muscularis propria; MAC C1, 2, or 3 imply nodal involvement along with extension into or through the bowel wall; MAC D means evidence of distant metastases. These correspond roughly to Duke's A, B, C and D. The AJCC or TMN classification defines stages 0 (carcinoma in situ) through IV.

SKIN CANCER
MELANOMA

The severity of melanoma is primarily related to the thickness of the primary lesion and to the presence of histologic ulceration. The American Joint Commission on Cancer's Stage Grouping for melanoma reflects these parameters. The T or tumor size component for identifiable melanomas is up to 1.0 mm thick for T1, 1.01 to 2.0 mm for T2, 2.01 to 4.0 mm for T3, and greater than 4.0 mm thick for T4. Within each of these groups for cases of melanoma in situ, an *a* is added for no ulceration and a *b* is added to indicate ulceration. Regional lymph node involvement is described by an N followed by a 1, 2 or 3 (for 1, 2-3, or 4 or more involved lymph nodes) and an *a* or *b* to indicate either micro- or macrometastases. Distant metastases, if present, are classified as M1a, b, or c, depending on the site. As with other schemes, an *X* after the letter indicates inability to assess, and a zero means no evidence. Staging is from 0 (in situ) to stage IV (distant metastases). Stages I and II have no nodal or metastatic involvement, and stage III means regional lymph node presence. Within each stage (I, II, and III) there are various subgroups, and the presence of ulceration can put a thinner melanoma in the same stage with a thicker but non-ulcerated lesion.

NONMELANOMA SKIN CANCERS

About four out of every five cases of nonmelanoma skin cancer are **basal cell carcinoma** (BCC), which usually presents as either a reddish ulcerated bump on the skin or as a lighter hardened plaque. Most other nonmelanoma skin cancers are **squamous cell carcinomas** (SCC), which usually appear as raised areas that are either red or skin-toned and have ulcerations and patchy areas of hard horny tissue called keratoses.

Organ transplant patients are prone to develop SCC. Patients with SCC are more likely to develop metastases than those with BCC, although the latter can reoccur at the primary site. Lack of differentiation in either type can portend a more clinically aggressive tumor. There are other generally rare and often more aggressive malignancies that can emulate BCC or SCC that should be excluded via differential diagnosis such as sebaceous gland carcinoma and Merkel cell carcinoma.

TUMOR LYSIS SYNDROME

Tumor lysis syndrome occurs when intracellular contents are released from tumor cells, leading to electrolyte imbalances (hyperkalemia, hyperphosphatemia, hypocalcemia, and hyperuricemia) when the kidneys are unable to excrete the large volume of metabolites. **Tumor lysis syndrome** is most common after treatment of hematologic malignancies but can occur due to any type of tumor that is sensitive to chemotherapy. The primary goals of therapy for tumor lysis syndrome are to increase urine production through IV hydration in order to prevent renal failure and to decrease uric acid concentration, usually with administration of allopurinol. The urine pH should be maintained at 7 or higher. Electrolyte levels should be closely monitored, as hyperkalemia is a risk. Patients at moderate risk (intermediate grade lymphomas, acute leukemias) should begin prophylactic allopurinol before chemotherapy, and those at higher risk (high grade lymphomas or acute leukemias with WBC count >50,000) should begin rasburicase.

Integumentary Pathophysiology

CELLULITIS

Cellulitis occurs when an area of the skin becomes infected, usually following injury or trauma to the skin. Cellulitis is most likely to be caused by staphylococcus or streptococcus bacteria. Patients with peripheral vascular disease, diabetes mellitus, and immunosuppression are at a higher risk for the development of cellulitis. **Signs and symptoms** include pain, erythema, and warmth at the affected site that progresses rapidly. In addition, the patient may experience fever, chills, fatigue, and malaise. **Diagnosis** is made by physical exam. Labs include complete blood count, culture of the involved area and blood. **Treatment** for cellulitis is the administration of antibiotics. Surgical irrigation and debridement may be indicated in severe cases.

SEPTIC ARTHRITIS

Septic arthritis is defined as an invasion of the joint space by bacteria, virus, or fungi. Elderly patients, immunosuppressed patients, and those with prosthetic joints are at an increased risk for septic arthritis. The most commonly affected joints include the knee, hip, shoulder, ankle, and wrist. **Signs and symptoms** include joint pain, fever, impaired range of motion, chills, edema, erythema, warmth, and the abnormal presence of fluid (effusion) surrounding the joint. **Diagnosis** is made by aspiration of the fluid with stain and culture, x-ray, and blood tests including CBC and cultures. **Treatment** is the administration of antibiotics. Surgical irrigation and debridement may also be indicated. The patient will likely undergo physical therapy as part of their recovery to improve and restore mobility and range of motion.

TISSUE DAMAGE RELATED TO ALLERGIC CONTACT DERMATITIS

Contact dermatitis is a localized response to contact with an allergen, resulting in a rash that may blister and itch. Common allergens include poison oak, poison ivy, latex, benzocaine, nickel, and preservatives, but there is a wide range of items, preparations, and products to which people may react.

Treatment includes:

- Identifying the causative agent through evaluating the area of the body affected, careful history, or skin patch testing to determine allergic responses
- Corticosteroids to control inflammation and itching
- Soothing oatmeal baths
- Pramoxine lotion to relieve itching
- Antihistamines to reduce allergic response
- Lesions should be gently cleansed and observed for signs of secondary infection
- Antibiotics are used only for secondary infections as indicated
- Rash is usually left open to dry
- Avoidance of allergen to prevent recurrence

Pressure Ulcers

Pressure ulcers occur when pressure from the weight of the body causes a decrease in perfusion, affecting arterial and capillary blood flow and resulting ischemia. Ulcers may then develop from pressure, shearing and friction. Common pressure points include the occiput, scapula, sacrum, buttocks, ischium, and heels. Patients with a decreased level of consciousness, brain/spinal cord injuries, peripheral neuropathies, malnutrition, dehydration, PVD, or impaired mobility are at a higher risk for pressure ulcers. Critically ill patients are at an increased risk due to prolonged immobility, sedation, and often incontinence of urine and stool. In addition, patients on vasopressors are at a higher risk due to the constriction of the peripheral circulation.

Signs and symptoms: Early stages include redness, tenderness, and firmness at the site of the ulcer. Once the ulcer progresses to severe tissue injury, bone, muscle, or tendons may be exposed, and there may be a yellow or black wound base in addition to pain and drainage at the site.

Diagnostics: Skin and wound assessment including staging of the ulcer.

Treatment: Wet-to-Dry dressings, Wound VAC® therapy, and hyperbaric oxygen may be used; a wound care consult is often advised.

Prevention: Begins with a risk assessment; the Braden scale is a commonly used scale. A score of 16 or below indicates that the patient is at risk. At-risk patients or patients with active ulcers should be placed on a turning and positioning schedule or on a specialty bed to relieve pressure. Moisture barriers and skin protectants may also be utilized.

National Pressure Ulcer Advisory Panel Staging

Pressure ulcers result from pressure or pressure with shear and/or friction over bony prominences. The **National Pressure Ulcer Advisory Panel (NPUAP) stages** include:

- **Suspected deep tissue injury**: Skin discolored, intact or blood blister
- **Stage I**: Intact skin with non-blanching reddened area
- **Stage II**: Abrasion or blistered area without slough but with partial-thickness skin loss
- **Stage III**: Deep ulcer with exposed subcutaneous tissue; tunneling or undermining may be evident with or without slough
- **Stage IV**: Deep ulcer, full thickness, with necrosis into muscle, bone, tendons, and/or joints
- **Unstageable**: Eschar and/or slough prevents staging prior to debridement

Patients should be placed on pressure reducing support surfaces and turned at least every two hours, avoiding the area(s) with a pressure ulcer. Wound care depends on the stage of the wound and the amount of drainage, but includes irrigation, debridement when necessary, antibiotics for infection, and appropriate dressing. Patients should be encouraged to have adequate protein and iron in their diets to promote healing and to maintain adequate hydration.

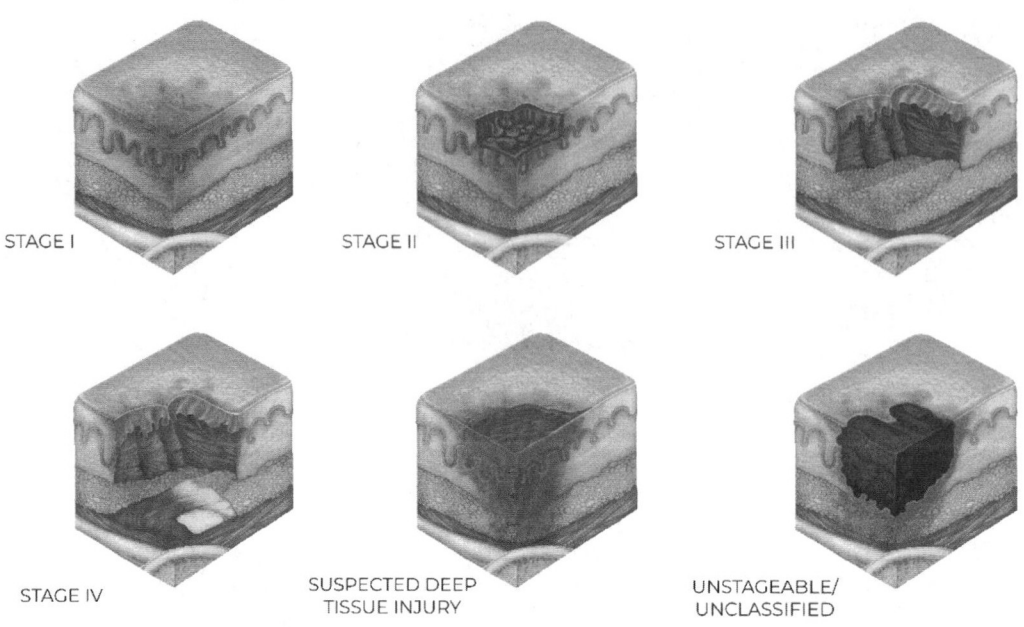

Infectious Wounds

All types of wounds have the potential to become infected. Infectious wounds are commonly health care acquired. Wound infections increase a patient's risk of sepsis, multisystem organ failure and death. Trauma patients are at an increased risk of developing an infected wound due to exposure to various contaminants that they may have encountered during their injury (e.g., dirt from a motor vehicle accident).

Signs and symptoms: Erythema, edema, induration, drainage, increasing pain and tenderness, fever, leukocytosis, and lymphangitis.

Diagnosis: Wound infections are diagnosed by wound cultures (anaerobic and aerobic). Fluid or tissue biopsy may also be performed.

Treatment: Wound infections are treated with antibiotics and a wound care regimen that includes routine cleaning and dressing of the wound. Wound care treatment is based on the type and severity of the wound. Surgical irrigation and debridement may also be indicated. For deep, complex wounds, a wound-care consult is often indicated.

Tissue Damage

Abrasion is damage to superficial layers of skin, such as with road burn or ligature marks.

Contusion occurs when friction or pressure causes damage to underlying vessels, resulting in bruising. Contusions that are bright red/purple with clear margins have occurred within 48 hours and those with receding edges or yellow-brown discoloration are older than 48 hours.

Laceration is a tear in the skin resulting from blunt force, often from falls on protuberances, such as elbows, or other blunt trauma. Lacerations may be partial to full-thickness.

Avulsion is tissue that is separated from its base and lost or without adequate base for attachment.

Treatments include:

- Local anesthetic if needed
- Low pressure, high volume irrigation with 35-50 mL syringe of open wound with normal saline, water, or non-antiseptic nonionic surfactants, and mechanical scrubbing of surrounding tissue with disinfectant
- Topical antibiotics as indicated
- Prophylactic antibiotics or antibiotic irrigation if wound contaminated
- Suturing/debridement as needed
- Hydrocolloids, Steri-Strips, and transparent dressings to stabilize flaps

Integumentary Procedures and Interventions

WOUND VACS

Wound vacuum-assisted closure (wound VAC) (AKA negative pressure wound therapy) uses subatmospheric (negative) pressure with a suction unit and a semi-occlusion vapor-permeable dressing. The suction reduces periwound and interstitial edema, decompressing vessels, improving circulation, stimulating production of new cells, and decreasing colonization of bacteria. Wound VAC also increases the rate of granulation and re-epithelialization to hasten healing. The wound must be debrided of necrotic tissue prior to treatment. Wound VAC is used for a variety of difficult-to-heal wounds, especially those that show less than 30% healing in 4 weeks of post-debridement treatment or those with excessive exudate, including chronic stage II and IV pressure ulcers, skin flaps, diabetic ulcer, acute wounds, burns, surgical wound, and those with dehiscence and nonresponsive arterial and venous ulcers. Contraindications include:

- Wound malignancy
- Untreated osteomyelitis
- Exposed blood vessels or organs
- Non-enteric, unexplored fistulas.

Nonadherent porous foam is cut to fit and cover the wound and is secured with occlusive transparent film with an opening cut to accommodate the drainage tube, which is attached to a suction canister in a closed system. The pressure should be set between 75 and 125 psi and the dressing changed 2 to 3 times weekly.

PRESSURE REDUCTION SURFACES

Pressure reduction surfaces redistribute pressure to prevent pressure ulcers and reduce shear and friction. There are various types of support surfaces for beds, examining tables, operating tables, and chairs. Functions of pressure reduction surfaces include temperature control, moisture control, and friction/shear control. **General use guidelines** include:

- Pressure redistribution support surfaces should be used for patients with stage II, III, and IV ulcers, as well as for those that are at-risk for developing pressure ulcers.
- Chairs should have gel or air support surfaces to redistribute pressure for chair bound patients, critically ill patients, or those who cannot move independently.

- Support surface material should provide at least an inch of support under areas to be protected when in use to prevent bottoming out. (Check by placing hand palm-up under the overlay below the pressure point.)
- Static support surfaces are appropriate for patients who can change position without increasing pressure to an ulcer.
- Dynamic support surfaces are needed for those who need assistance to move or when static pressure devices provide less than an inch of support.

Musculoskeletal Pathophysiology

IMMOBILITY

Critical care patients are often **immobile** for extended periods of time, thereby increasing their risk of skin breakdown and the development of pressure ulcers, deep vein thrombosis, functional decline, decreased muscle mass, impaired coordination and gait, cardiovascular deconditioning, depression, and constipation. Immobility leads to impaired physical functioning in which muscle mass is lost and weakness develops. Intensive care unit acquired weakness can develop during hospitalization and is associated with an increased hospital length of stay as well as an increased mortality rate. ICU acquired weakness may last years after discharge with residual effects often affecting the patient's quality of life. Progressive mobility is defined as the gradual progression of positioning and mobility techniques and should be utilized to improve muscle strength and provide the patient a greater ability to resume activities of daily living. Patients should be assessed daily for their readiness to progress in their mobility goals in order to prevent the adverse effects of immobility.

GAIT DISORDERS

Functional movement disorders are defined as an involuntary, abnormal movement of part of the body in which pathophysiology is not fully understood. Functional tremors are the most frequent type of functional movement disorder. Dystonia, myoclonus, and Parkinsonism are other types of functional movement disorders. Functional gait disorders are another type of functional movement disorder and are common in the elderly. Gait disorders can manifest as a dragging gait, knee buckling, small slow steps or "walking on ice," swaying gait, fluctuating gait, hesitant gait, and hyperkinetic gait in which there is excessive movement of the arms, trunk, and legs when ambulating. Patients with gait disorders are at an increased risk of falling. Gait disorders are diagnosed by a thorough clinical examination (including a neurologic assessment) and health history. Treatment for functional gait disorders includes strength and balance training. Assistive devices such as walkers and canes may also be utilized.

FALLS

Falls are the most commonly occurring adverse event in the hospital setting. Confusion and agitation are factors that contribute to an increased risk for falling. In addition, impaired balance or gait, orthostatic hypotension, altered mobility, a history of falling, advanced age and the use of certain medications are additional risk factors. Approximately 30% of patient falls result in injury, some of which can significantly contribute to an increase in morbidity and mortality including fractures and subdural hematomas. Both physical and environmental factors contribute to patient falls, some of which are preventable. Fall prevention strategies include utilization of a standardized fall risk assessment to determine the patient's level of risk and subsequent care planning and interventions individualized to the patient. Fall prevention should also be balanced with progressive mobility. Many falls are related to toileting needs, and nurses often utilize scheduled rounding to address such needs.

Carpal Tunnel Syndrome

Carpal tunnel syndrome is a type of entrapment neuropathy in which the median nerve is compressed by thickening of the flexor tendon sheath, skeletal encroachment, or mass in the soft tissue. Carpal tunnel syndrome is often associated with repetitive hand activities, arthritis, hypothyroidism, diabetes, and pregnancy. Patients complain of pain in wrist, radiating to forearm, and numbness and tingling in the first 2 to 3 fingers, especially during the night.

Diagnosis is based on symptoms and tests such as:

- **Positive Tinel test**: Gentle percussion over medial nerve in inner aspect of wrist elicits numbness and pain.
- **Positive Phalen test**: The backs of the hands are pressed together and the wrists sharply flexed for 1 minute to elicit pain and numbness.

Treatment includes identifying and treating the underlying cause:

- Steroid injection may relieve symptoms
- Splint during the night or during repetitive activities
- Modification of activities
- Referral for decompression surgery in recalcitrant cases or those with severe loss of sensation

Infectious Arthritis

Infectious arthritis may be bacterial, viral (rubella, parvovirus, and hepatitis B), parasitic, or fungal, with bacterial arthritis causing the most rapid destruction to the joint. *Neisseria gonorrhoeae* (most common), *Staphylococcus*, *Streptococcus*, and *Escherichia coli* are the most common bacterial agents. The infection may be bloodborne or spread from an infection near the joint or from direct implantation or postoperative contamination of the wound. Usually, the infection involves just one joint.

Symptoms include acute edema, erythema, and pain in a joint. Systemic reactions, such as fever and polyarthralgia, may occur, especially with gonorrhea.

Diagnosis requires a complete history and physical examination, arthrocentesis and synovial fluid culture, and WBC.

Treatment includes:

- Antibiotics as indicated by organism
- Arthrocentesis to drain fluid accumulation in joint (may need to be repeated)
- Analgesia

Bursitis and Tendinitis

Bursitis is inflammation of the bursa, fluid-filled spaces or sacs that form in tissues to reduce friction, causing thickening of the lining of the bursal walls. This can be the result of infection, trauma, crystal deposits, or chronic friction from trauma.

Tendinitis is inflammation of the long, tubular tendons and tendon sheaths adjacent to the bursa. Causes of tendinitis are similar to bursitis but tendinitis may also be caused by quinolone antibiotics. Frequently, both bursa and tendons are inflamed. Common types of bursitis include shoulder, olecranon (elbow), trochanteric (hip), and prepatellar (front of knee). Common types of tendinitis include wrist, Achilles, patellar, and rotator cuff.

Symptoms include pain with movement, edema, dysfunction, and decreased range of motion.

Diagnosis is by clinical examination, although x-rays may rule out fractures. The bursa may be aspirated diagnostically to aid in ruling out other diagnosis, like gout or infection.

Treatment for bursitis and tendinitis includes:

- Rest and immobilization
- NSAIDs
- Application of cold packs to affected area
- Steroid injections

JOINT EFFUSION AND ARTHROCENTESIS

Joint effusion is the accumulation of fluid (clear, bloody, or purulent) within a joint capsule. Joint effusion can cause pressure on the joint and severe pain. Arthrocentesis relieves the pressure and the fluid aspirated can be examined to aid in diagnosis. Arthrocentesis is usually contraindicated in the presence of overlying infection, prosthetic joint, and coagulopathy without referral to an orthopedic specialist.

Procedure:

1. Patient is **positioned** according to joint to be aspirated and encouraged to relax muscles.
2. **Overlying area** is cleansed with povidone-iodine solution, air-dried a few minutes, and cleansed of iodine with alcohol wipe.
3. **Local anesthetic** is given to the area (but not into the joint) with 25- to 30-gauge needle (lidocaine 1-2%) or a regional nerve block for severe pain.
4. The joint is **aspirated** with insertion in a straight line, using a 30-60 mL syringe (depending upon expected amount of fluid) and an 18- to 22-gauge needle or IV catheter.
5. The joint is completely **drained** of fluid.
6. Observe for **complications**: bleeding, infection, or allergic reaction.

LUMBOSACRAL PAIN

Lumbosacral (low back) pain may be related to strain, muscular weakness, osteoarthritis, spinal stenosis, herniated disks, vertebral fractures, bony metastasis, infection, or other musculoskeletal disorders. Disk herniation or other joint changes put pressure on nerves leaving the spinal cord, causing pain to radiate along the nerve. Pain may be acute or chronic (more than 3 months).

Symptoms include local or pain radiating down the leg (radiculopathy), impaired gait and reflexes, difference in leg lengths, decreased motor strength, and alteration of sensation, including numbness.

Diagnosis is by careful clinical examination and history as well as x-ray (fractures, scoliosis, dislocations), CT (identifies underlying problems), MRI (spinal pathology), and/or EMG and nerve conduction studies. Diagnostic studies may be deferred in many cases for 4-6 weeks as symptoms may resolve over time. **Treatments** for nonspecific back pain include:

- Analgesia: acetaminophen, NSAIDS, opiates
- Encourage activity to tolerance but not bed rest

- Muscle relaxants: diazepam 5-10 mg every 6-8 hours
- Cold and heat compresses

STRAINS AND SPRAINS

A **strain** is an overstretching of a part of the musculature ("pulled muscle") that causes microscopic tears in the muscle, usually resulting from excess stress or overuse of the muscle. Onset of pain is usually sudden with local tenderness on use of the muscle. A **sprain** is damage to a joint, with a partial rupture of the supporting ligaments, usually caused by wrenching or twisting that may occur with a fall. The rupture can damage blood vessels, resulting in edema, tenderness at the joint, and pain on movement with pain increasing over 2-3 hours after injury. An avulsion fracture (bone fragment pulled away by a ligament) may occur with strain, so x-rays rule out fractures.

Treatment for both strains and sprains includes:

- **RICE protocol**: rest, ice, compression, and elevation
- **Ice compresses** (wet or dry) applied 20-30 minutes intermittently for 48 hours and then intermittent heat 15-20 minutes 3-4 times daily
- Monitor **neurovascular status** (especially for sprain)
- **Immobilization** as indicated for sprains for 1-3 weeks

OSTEOMYELITIS

Musculoskeletal infections encompass a variety of different disorders with differing pathologies. Osteomyelitis, cellulitis, and septic arthritis are examples of musculoskeletal infections that can be both serious and debilitating in nature.

Osteomyelitis is an infection of the bone that can occur from an open fracture or an infection that has occurred somewhere else in the body. Osteomyelitis can also be caused by wounds or soft tissue infections that have progressed and extended to the bone. Signs and symptoms of osteomyelitis include pain, swelling, erythema and possible drainage at the site. The patient may also experience fever and chills. Diagnosis includes lab work including a complete blood count, erythrocyte sedimentation rate (ESR), C-reactive protein (CRP), and blood cultures, as well as radiologic testing that may include CT, MRI, X-ray, bone scan, or a bone biopsy. Treatment includes the administration of IV antibiotics. A needle aspiration may be performed to determine the organism and drain the area. Surgical irrigation and debridement may also be indicated.

COMPARTMENT SYNDROME

Compartment syndrome occurs when there is an increase in the amount of pressure within a grouping of muscles, nerves, and blood vessels resulting in compromised blood flow to muscles and nerves. This is a medical emergency. If left untreated, tissue ischemia and eventual tissue death will occur. **Compartment syndrome** most often occurs after a fracture, particularly a long bone fracture, but can also occur with crushing syndrome and rhabdomyolysis. Risk factors include lower extremity trauma, massive tissue injury, venous obstruction, the use of certain medications (anticoagulants), burns and compressive dressings or casts. Compartment syndrome can affect the hand, forearm, upper arm, abdomen, and lower extremities. It can be acute or chronic in nature with acute compartment syndrome requiring immediate intervention.

Signs and symptoms: Intense pain, decreased sensation and paresthesia, firmness at the affected site, swelling and tightness at the affected site, pallor and pulselessness (late signs).

Diagnosis: Physical assessment and the measurement of intra-compartmental pressures.

Treatment: The goal of treatment in compartment syndrome is decompression and the restoration of perfusion to the affected area. Surgical fasciotomy is often indicated to relieve pressure and prevent tissue death. Fasciotomy involves the opening of the skin and muscle fascia to release the pressure within the compartment and restore blood flow to the area.

Prevention: Leave large abdominal wounds open to drain, delay casting on affected extremities, and use flexible casts. Watch circumferential burns closely and perform frequent neurovascular checks on those at risk.

Rhabdomyolysis

Rhabdomyolysis occurs when damage of the cells of the skeletal muscles causes the release of toxins from injured cells into the bloodstream. Rhabdomyolysis may be caused by trauma, tissue ischemia, infection, certain medications (statins, selective serotonin reuptake inhibitors, lithium, and antihistamines), sepsis, immobilization, extraordinary physical exertion, myopathies and cocaine or alcohol abuse. Additionally, rhabdomyolysis may occur with exposure to certain toxins such as snake/insect venoms or mushroom poisoning. In rare circumstances, the identifiable cause cannot be determined. The most serious complication of rhabdomyolysis is renal failure. Rhabdomyolysis may be life threatening. Early recognition and treatment are critical to avoid serious complications and for patients to make a full recovery.

Signs and symptoms: Electrolyte imbalance, muscle pain and weakness, fever, tachycardia, dehydration, fatigue, lethargy, hypotension, and metabolic acidosis. Dark, reddish-brown urine may occur due to the presence of myoglobin released from the muscles and excreted into the urine.

Diagnosis: Laboratory studies such as creatinine kinase (CK) level, metabolic panel, urinalysis, and blood gases.

Treatment: The treatment of rhabdomyolysis includes fluid administration to eliminate toxins and prevent renal failure. Bicarbonate may be administered to correct metabolic acidosis. Mannitol or dopamine may be administered to increase renal perfusion. Electrolyte replacement may also be indicated. In severe cases, emergency dialysis may be necessary.

Multisystem Pathophysiology

Range of Severe Infection

There are a number of terms used to refer to severe infections which are often used interchangeably. It is important to know these terms to properly perform the continuum of care.

- **Bacteremia** is the presence of bacteria in the blood without systemic infection.
- **Septicemia** is a systemic infection caused by pathogens (usually bacteria or fungi) present in the blood.
- **Systemic inflammatory response syndrome** (SIRS) is a generalized inflammatory response affecting many organ systems. It may be caused by infectious or non-infectious agents, such as trauma, burns, adrenal insufficiency, pulmonary embolism, and drug overdose. If an infectious agent is identified or suspected, SIRS is an aspect of sepsis. Infective agents include a wide range of bacteria and fungi, including *Streptococcus pneumoniae* and *Staphylococcus aureus*. SIRS includes 2 of the following:
    - Elevated (>38 °C) or subnormal rectal temperature (<36 °C)
    - Tachypnea or $PaCO_2$ <32 mmHg
    - Tachycardia

- o Leukocytosis (>12,000) or leukopenia (<4000)
- **Sepsis** is the presence of infection either locally or systemically in which there is a generalized life-threatening inflammatory response (SIRS). It includes all the indications for SIRS as well as one of the following:
  - o Changes in mental status
  - o Hypoxemia without preexisting pulmonary disease
  - o Elevation in plasma lactate
  - o Decreased urinary output <5 mL/kg/hr for ≥1 hour
- **Severe sepsis** includes both indications of SIRS and sepsis as well as indications of increasing organ dysfunction with inadequate perfusion and/or hypotension.
- **Septic shock** is a progression from severe sepsis in which refractory hypotension occurs despite treatment. There may be indications of lactic acidosis.
- **Multi-organ dysfunction syndrome** (MODS) is the most common cause of sepsis-related death. Cardiac function becomes depressed, acute respiratory distress syndrome (ARDS) may develop, and renal failure may follow acute tubular necrosis or cortical necrosis. Thrombocytopenia appears in about 30% of those affected and may result in disseminated intravascular coagulation (DIC). Liver damage and bowel necrosis may occur.

SHOCK

There are a number of different types of shock, but there are general characteristics that they have in common. In all types of shock, there is a marked decrease in tissue perfusion related to hypotension, so that there is insufficient oxygen delivered to the tissues and inadequate removal of cellular waste products, causing injury to tissue:

- Hypotension (systolic below 90 mmHg); this may be somewhat higher (110 mmHg) in those who are initially hypertensive
- Decreased urinary output (<0.5 mL/kg/hr), especially marked in hypovolemic shock
- Metabolic acidosis
- Peripheral/cutaneous vasoconstriction/vasodilation resulting in cool, clammy skin
- Alterations in level of consciousness

Types of shock are as follows:

- **Distributive:** Preload decreased, CO increased, SVR decreased
- **Cardiogenic:** Preload increased, CO decreased, SVR increased
- **Hypovolemic:** Preload decreased, CO decreased, SVR increased

SEPTIC SHOCK

Septic shock is caused by toxins produced by bacteria and cytokines that the body produces in response to severe infection, resulting in a complex syndrome of disorders. **Symptoms** are wide-ranging:

- **Initial**: Hyper- or hypothermia, increased temperature (>38 °C) with chills, tachycardia with increased pulse pressure, tachypnea, alterations in mental status (dullness), hypotension, hyperventilation with respiratory alkalosis ($PaCO_2$ ≤30 mmHg), increased lactic acid, unstable BP, and dehydration with increased urinary output
- **Cardiovascular**: Myocardial depression and dysrhythmias
- **Respiratory**: Acute respiratory distress syndrome (ARDS)
- **Renal**: Acute kidney injury (AKI) with decreased urinary output and increased BUN

- **Hepatic**: Jaundice and liver dysfunction with an increase in transaminase, alkaline phosphatase, and bilirubin
- **Hematologic**: Mild or severe blood loss (from mucosal ulcerations), neutropenia or neutrophilia, decreased platelets, and DIC
- **Endocrine**: Hyperglycemia, hypoglycemia (rare)
- **Skin**: Cellulitis, erysipelas, and fasciitis, acrocyanotic and necrotic peripheral lesions

DIAGNOSIS AND TREATMENT

Septic shock is most common in newborns, those >50, and those who are immunocompromised. There is no specific test to confirm a diagnosis of septic shock, so **diagnosis** is based on clinical findings and tests that evaluate hematologic, infectious, and metabolic states: Lactic acid, CBC, DIC panel, electrolytes, liver function tests, BUN, creatinine, blood glucose, ABGs, urinalysis, ECG, radiographs, blood and urine cultures.

Treatment must be aggressive and includes:

- Oxygen and endotracheal intubation as necessary
- IV access with 2-large bore catheters and central venous line
- Rapid fluid administration at 0.5L NS or isotonic crystalloid every 5-10 minutes as needed (to 4-6 L)
- Monitoring urinary output to optimal >30 mL/hr (>0.5-1 mL/kg/hr)
- Inotropic or vasoconstrictive agents (dopamine, dobutamine, norepinephrine) if no response to fluids or fluid overload
- Empiric IV antibiotic therapy (usually with 2 broad spectrum antibiotics for both gram-positive and gram-negative bacteria) until cultures return and antibiotics may be changed
- Hemodynamic and laboratory monitoring
- Removing source of infection (abscess, catheter)

DISTRIBUTIVE SHOCK

Distributive shock occurs with adequate blood volume but inadequate intravascular volume because of arterial/venous dilation that results in decreased vascular tone and hypoperfusion of internal organs. Cardiac output may be normal or blood may pool, decreasing cardiac output. **Distributive shock** may result from anaphylactic shock, septic shock, neurogenic shock, and drug ingestions.

Symptoms include:

- Hypotension (systolic <90 mmHg or <40 mmHg below normal), tachypnea, tachycardia (>90) (may be lower if patient receiving β-blockers)
- Hypoxemia
- Skin initially warm, later hypoperfused
- Hyper- or hypothermia (>38 °C or <36 °C)
- Alterations in mentation
- Decreased urinary output
- Symptoms related to underlying cause

Treatment includes:

- Treating underlying cause while stabilizing hemodynamics
- Oxygen with endotracheal intubation if necessary

- Rapid fluid administration at 0.25-0.5 L NS or isotonic crystalloid every 5-10 minutes as needed to 2-3 L
- Vasoconstrictive and inotropic agents (dopamine, dobutamine, norepinephrine) if necessary, for patients with profound hypotension

NEUROGENIC SHOCK

Neurogenic shock is a type of distributive shock that occurs when injury to the CNS from trauma resulting in acute spinal cord injury (from both blunt and penetrating injuries), neurological diseases, drugs, or anesthesia, impairs the autonomic nervous system that controls the cardiovascular system. The degree of symptoms relates to the level of injury with injuries above T1 capable of causing disruption of the entire sympathetic nervous system and lower injuries causing various degrees of disruption. Even incomplete spinal cord injury can cause neurogenic shock.

Symptoms include:

- Hypotension and warm dry skin related to lack of vascular tone that results in hypothermia from loss of cutaneous heat
- Bradycardia (common but not universal)

Treatment includes:

- ABCDE (airway, breathing, circulation, disability evaluation, exposure)
- Rapid fluid administration with crystalloid to keep mean arterial pressure at 85-90 mmHg
- Placement of pulmonary artery catheter to monitor fluid overload
- Inotropic agents (dopamine, dobutamine) if fluids don't correct hypotension
- Atropine for persistent bradycardia

ANAPHYLACTIC SHOCK

Anaphylactic reaction or anaphylactic shock may present with a few symptoms or a wide range of potentially lethal effects.

Symptoms may recur after the initial treatment (biphasic anaphylaxis), so careful monitoring is essential:

- Sudden onset of weakness, dizziness, confusion
- Severe generalized edema and angioedema; lips and tongue may swell
- Urticaria
- Increased permeability of vascular system and loss of vascular tone leading to severe hypotension and shock
- Laryngospasm/bronchospasm with obstruction of airway causing dyspnea and wheezing
- Nausea, vomiting, and diarrhea
- Seizures, coma, and death

Treatments:

- Establish patent airway and intubate if necessary, for ventilation
- Provide oxygen at 100% high flow
- Monitor VS
- Administer epinephrine (Epi-pen® or solution)
- Albuterol per nebulizer for bronchospasm

- Intravenous fluids to provide bolus of fluids for hypotension
- Diphenhydramine if shock persists
- Methylprednisolone if no response to other drugs

Hypovolemic Shock/Volume Deficit

Hypovolemic shock occurs when there is inadequate intravascular fluid. The loss may be *absolute* because of an internal shifting of fluid or an external loss of fluid, as occurs with massive hemorrhage, thermal injuries, severe vomiting or diarrhea, and internal injuries (such as ruptured spleen or dissecting arteries) that interfere with intravascular integrity. Hypovolemia may also be *relative* and related to vasodilation, increased capillary membrane permeability from sepsis or injuries, and decreased colloidal osmotic pressure that may occur with loss of sodium and some disorders, such as hypopituitarism and cirrhosis.

Hypovolemic shock is **classified** according to the degree of fluid loss:

- **Class I:** <750 mL or ≤15% of total circulating volume (TCV)
- **Class II:** 750-1500 mL or 15-30% of TCV
- **Class III:** 1500-2000 mL or 30-40% of TCV
- **Class IV:** >2000 mL or >40% of TCV

Symptoms and Treatment

Hypovolemic shock occurs when the total circulating volume of fluid decreases, leading to a fall in venous return that in turn causes a decrease in ventricular filling and preload, indicated by ↓ in right atrial pressure (RAP) and pulmonary artery occlusion pressure (PAOP). This results in a decrease in stroke volume and cardiac output. This in turn causes generalized arterial vasoconstriction, increasing afterload (↑ systemic vascular resistance), causing decreased tissue perfusion.

Symptoms: Anxiety, pallor, cool and clammy skin, delayed capillary refill, cyanosis, hypotension, increasing respirations, weak, thready pulse.

Treatment is aimed at identifying and treating the cause:

- Administration of blood, blood products, autotransfusion, colloids (such as plasma protein fraction), and/or crystalloids (such as normal saline)
- Oxygen; intubation and ventilation may be necessary
- Medications may include vasopressors, such as dopamine. NOTE: Fluids must be given before starting vasopressors!

Toxic Exposures
Carbon Monoxide Poisoning

Carbon monoxide (CO) poisoning occurs with inhalation of fossil fuel exhausts from engines, emission of gas or coal heaters, indoor use of charcoal, and smoke and fumes. The CO binds with hemoglobin, preventing oxygen carriage and impairing oxygen delivery to tissue.

Diagnosis includes history, on-site oximetry reports, neurological examination, and CO neuropsychological screening battery (CONSB) done with patient breathing room air, CBC, electrolytes, ABGs, ECG, chest radiograph (for dyspnea); *pulse oximetry is not accurate in these patients*.

Symptoms:

- Cardiac: chest pain, palpitations, decreased capillary refill, hypotension, and cardiac arrest
- CNS: malaise, nausea, vomiting, lethargy, stroke, coma, and seizure
- Secondary injuries: Rhabdomyolysis, AKI, non-cardiogenic pulmonary edema, multiple organ failure (MOF), DIC, and encephalopathy

Treatment includes:

- Immediate support of airway, breathing, and circulation
- Non-barometric oxygen (100%) by non-breathing mask with reservoir or ETT if necessary
- Mild: Continue oxygen for 4 hours with reassessment
- Severe: hyperbaric oxygen therapy (usually 3 treatments) to improve oxygen delivery

CYANIDE POISONING

Cyanide poisoning, from hydrogen cyanide (HCN) or cyanide salts, can result from sodium nitroprusside infusions, inhalation of burning plastics, intentional or accidental ingestion or dermal exposure, occupation exposure, ingestion of some plant products, and the manufacture of PCP. Inhalation of HCN causes immediate symptoms, and the ingestion of cyanide salts causes symptoms within minutes.

Diagnosis is by history, clinical examination, normal PaO_2 and metabolic acidosis.

Symptoms: Increase in severity and alter with the amount of exposure: tachycardia, hypertension, leading to bradycardia, hypotension, and cardiac arrest. Pink or cherry-colored skin because of oxygen remaining in the blood. Other symptoms include headaches, lethargy, seizures, coma, dyspnea, tachypnea, and respiratory arrest.

Treatment includes:

- Supportive care as indicated
- Removal of contaminated clothes
- Gastric decontamination
- Copious irrigation for topical exposure
- Antidotes:
    - Amyl nitrate ampule cracked and inhaled 30 seconds
    - Sodium nitrite (3%) 10 mL IV
    - Sodium thiosulfate (25%) 50 mL IV

CAUSTIC INGESTIONS

Caustic ingestions of acids (pH <7) such as sulfuric, acetic, hydrochloric, and hydrofluoric found in many cleaning agents and alkalis (pH >7) such as sodium hydroxide, potassium hydroxide, sodium tripolyphosphate (in detergents) and sodium hypochlorite (bleach) can result in severe injury and death. Acids cause coagulation necrosis in the esophagus and stomach and may result in metabolic acidosis, hemolysis, and renal failure if systemically absorbed. Alkali injuries cause liquefaction necrosis, resulting in deeper ulcerations, often of the esophagus, but may involve perforation and abdominal necrosis with multi-organ damage.

Diagnosis is by detailed history, airway examination (oral intubation if possible), arterial blood gas, electrolytes, CBC, hepatic and coagulation tests, radiograph, and CT for perforations.

Symptoms may vary but can include pain, dyspnea, oral burns, dysphonia, and vomiting.

Treatment includes:

- Supportive and symptomatic therapy
- <u>NO</u> ipecac, charcoal, neutralization, or dilution
- NG tube for acids only to aspirate residual
- Endoscopy in first few hours to evaluate injury/perforations
- Sodium bicarbonate for pH <7.10
- Prednisolone (alkali injuries)

ALLERGIC REACTIONS

Exposure to certain toxins, medications, illegal substances, and allergens can cause life threatening effects in some patients. The physiologic response of the patient is dependent on the agent and the degree of exposure. Tissue hypoperfusion and lactic acidosis often occur as a result of the exposure. This can lead to metabolic acidosis, shock, organ failure, and death.

Signs and symptoms: In allergic type reactions, urticaria, pruritus, chest, back or abdominal pain, facial flushing, shortness of breath, wheezing and stridor may occur. Beta- and alpha-adrenergic responses may occur with exposure to amphetamines, cocaine, ephedrine, and pseudoephedrine. This response is manifested by diaphoresis, hypertension, tachycardia, and mydriasis. Diarrhea, nausea, and vomiting can occur with exposure to certain toxins.

Diagnosis: Physical assessment and testing to discover the toxin, drug, or allergen the patient was exposed to. Labs—blood gases, BMP, complete blood count, toxicology screen, urinalysis, and allergy testing.

Treatment: Priority is to eliminate exposure to the drug/toxin/allergen. Antidotes (if available) may be administered in the case of toxin exposure. Activated charcoal may be administered in the case of medication/drug overdose. For allergic reactions, antihistamines and corticosteroids may be administered. Severe allergic reactions may need to be treated with epinephrine. Dialysis may be indicated in some patients. Sodium bicarbonate may be administered for the treatment of metabolic acidosis caused by many toxic reactions.

ACETAMINOPHEN TOXICITY

Acetaminophen toxicity from accidental or intentional overdose has high rates of morbidity and mortality unless promptly treated. **Diagnosis** is by history and acetaminophen level, which should be completed within 8 hours of ingestion if possible. Toxicity occurs with dosage >140 mg/kg in one dose or >7.5g in 24 hours.

Symptoms occur in stages:

1. (Initial) Minor gastrointestinal upset
2. (Days 2-3) Hepatotoxicity with RUQ pain and increased AST, ALT, and bilirubin
3. (Days 3-4) Hepatic failure with metabolic acidosis, coagulopathy, renal failure, encephalopathy, nausea, vomiting, and possible death
4. (Days 5-12) Recovery period for survivors

Treatment includes:

- GI decontamination with activated charcoal (orally or NG) <24 hours
- Toxicity is plotted on the Rumack-Matthew nomogram with serum levels >150 requiring antidote. The antidote is most effective ≤8 hours of ingestion but decreases hepatotoxicity even >24 hours.
- Antidote: 72-hour N-acetylcysteine (NAC) protocol includes 140 mg/kg initially and 70 mg/kg every 4 hours for 17 more doses (orally or IV)
- Supportive therapy: Continuous dialysis, fluids, blood pressure medications

AMPHETAMINE AND COCAINE TOXICITY

Amphetamine toxicity may be caused by IV, inhalation, or insufflation of various substances that include methamphetamine (MDA or "ecstasy"), methylphenidate (Ritalin®), methylenedioxymethamphetamine (MDMA), and ephedrine and phenylpropanolamine. Cocaine may be ingested orally, IV or by insufflation while crack cocaine may be smoked. Amphetamines and cocaine are CNS stimulants that can cause multi-system abnormalities.

Symptoms may include chest pain, dysrhythmias, myocardial ischemia, MI, seizures, intracranial infarctions, hypertension, dystonia, repetitive movements, unilateral blindness, lethargy, rhabdomyolysis with acute kidney failure, perforated nasal septum (cocaine), and paranoid psychosis (amphetamines). Crack cocaine may cause pulmonary hemorrhage, asthma, pulmonary edema, barotrauma, and pneumothorax. Swallowing packs of cocaine can cause intestinal ischemia, colitis, necrosis, and perforation. **Diagnosis** includes clinical findings, CBC, chemistry panel, toxicology screening, ECG, and radiography.

Treatment includes:

- Gastric emptying (<1 hour). Charcoal administration
- IV access. Supplemental oxygen
- Sedation for seizures: Lorazepam 2 mg, diazepam 5 mg IV titrated in repeated doses
- Agitation: Haloperidol
- Hypertension: Nitroprusside/nicardipine, phentolamine IV
- Cocaine quinidine-like effects: Sodium bicarbonate

SALICYLATE TOXICITY

Salicylate toxicity may be acute or chronic and is caused by ingestion of OTC drugs containing salicylates, such as ASA, Pepto-Bismol®, and products used in hot inhalers.

Diagnosis is by ferric chloride or Ames Phenistix tests. Symptoms vary according to age and amount of ingestion. Co-ingestion of sedatives may alter symptoms.

Symptoms include:

- <150 mg/kg: Nausea and vomiting
- 150-300 mg/kg: Vomiting, hyperpnea, diaphoresis, tinnitus, and alterations in acid-base balance
- >300 mg/kg (usually intentional overdose): Nausea, vomiting, diaphoresis, tinnitus, hyperventilation, respiratory alkalosis, and metabolic acidosis
- Chronic toxicity results in hyperventilation, tremor, and papilledema, alterations in mental status, pulmonary edema, seizures, and coma

Treatment includes:

- Gastric decontamination with lavage (≤1 hour) and charcoal
- Volume replacement (D5W)
- Sodium bicarbonate 1-2 mEq/kg
- Monitoring of salicylate concentration, acid-base, and electrolytes every hour
- Whole-bowel irrigation (sustained release tablets)

BENZODIAZEPINE TOXICITY

Benzodiazepine toxicity may result from accidental or intentional overdose with such drugs as Xanax®, Librium®, Valium®, Ativan®, Serax®, Versed®, and Restoril®. Mortality is usually the result of co-ingestion of other drugs.

Diagnosis is based on history and clinical exam, as benzodiazepine level does not correlate well with toxicity.

Symptoms: Non-specific neurological changes: Lethargy, dizziness, alterations in consciousness, and ataxia. Respiratory depression and hypotension are rare complications. Coma and severe central nervous depression are usually caused by co-ingestions.

Treatment includes:

- Gastric emptying (<1 hour)
- Charcoal
- Concentrated dextrose, thiamine, and naloxone if co-ingestions suspected, especially with altered mental status
- Monitoring for CNS/respiratory depression
- Supportive care
- Flumazenil (antagonist) 0.2 mg each minute to total 3 mg may be used in some cases but not routinely advised because of complications related to benzodiazepine dependency or co-ingestion of cyclic antidepressants. Flumazenil is contraindicated in patients with increased ICP.

ETHANOL OVERDOSE

Ethanol overdose affects the central nervous system as well as other organs in the body. Alcohol is an inhibitory neurotransmitter that depresses the central nervous system. In most states, the legal intoxication blood alcohol level is defined as 100 mg/dL. Blood alcohol levels of **500 mg/dL or greater** are associated with a high mortality rate. The central nervous system depressant effect is further enhanced when alcohol is mixed with other agents.

Ethanol is absorbed through the mucosa of the mouth, stomach, and intestines, with concentrations peaking about 30-60 minutes after ingestion. If people are easily aroused, they can usually safely sleep off the effects of ingesting too much alcohol, but if the person is semi-conscious or unconscious, emergency medical treatment should be initiated.

Symptoms include:

- Altered mental status with slurred speech and stupor
- Nausea and vomiting
- Hypotension
- Bradycardia with arrhythmias

- Respiratory depression and hypoxia
- Cold, clammy skin or flushed skin (from vasodilation)
- Acute pancreatitis with abdominal pain
- Lack of consciousness
- Circulatory collapse

Treatment includes:

- Careful monitoring of arterial blood gases and oxygen saturation
- Ensure patent airway with intubation and ventilation if necessary
- Intravenous fluids
- Dextrose to correct hypoglycemia if indicated
- Maintain body temperature (warming blanket)
- Dialysis may be necessary in severe cases

GASTRIC EMPTYING FOR TOXIC SUBSTANCE INGESTION

Gastric emptying for toxic substance ingestion should be done ≤60 minutes of ingestion for large life-threatening amounts of poison. The patient requires IV access, oximetry, and cardiac monitoring. Sedation (1-2 mg IV midazolam) or rapid sequence induction and endotracheal intubation may be necessary. Patients should be positioned in left lateral decubitus position with head down at 20° to prevent passage of stomach contents into duodenum, although intubated patients may be lavaged in the supine position. With a bite block in place, an orogastric Y-tube (36-40 Fr. for adults) should be inserted after estimating length. Placement should be confirmed with injection of 50 mL of air confirmed under auscultation and aspiration of gastric contents, as well as abdominal x-ray (pH may not be reliable depending on substance ingested). Irrigation is done by gravity instillation of about 200-300 mL warmed (45 °C) tap water or NS. The instillation side is clamped and drainage side opened. This is repeated until fluid returns clear. A slurry of charcoal is then instilled, and the tube is clamped and removed when procedures completed.

HEAT-RELATED ILLNESS

Children and the elderly are particularly vulnerable to heat-related illness, especially when heat is combined with humidity. Heat-related illnesses occur when heat accumulation in the body outpaces dissipation, resulting in increased temperature and dehydration, which can then lead to thermoregulatory failure and multiple organ dysfunction syndromes. Each year in the United States, about 29 children die from heat stroke after being left in automobiles. At temperatures of 72-96 °F, the temperature in a car rises 3.2 °F every 5 minutes, with 80% of rise within 30 minutes. Temperatures can reach 117 °F even on cool days. There are three **types of heat-related illness**:

- **Heat stress**: Increased temperature causes dehydration. Patient may develop swelling of hands and feet, itching of skin, sunburn, heat syncope (pale moist skin, hypotension), heat cramps, and heat tetany (respiratory alkalosis). Treatment includes removing from heat, cooling, hydrating, and replacing sodium.
- **Heat exhaustion**: Involves water or sodium depletion, with sodium depletion common in patients who are not acclimated to heat. Heat exhaustion can result in flu-like aching, nausea and vomiting, headaches, dizziness, and hypotension with cold, clammy skin and diaphoresis. Temperature may be normal or elevated to less than 106 °F. Treatment to cool the body and replace sodium and fluids must be prompt in order to prevent heat stroke. Careful monitoring is important and reactions may be delayed.

- **Heat stroke**: Involves failure of the thermoregulatory system with temperatures that may be more than 106 °F and can result in seizures, neurological damage, multiple organ failures, and death. Exertional heat stroke often occurs in young athletes who engage in strenuous activities in high heat. Young children are susceptible to nonexertional heat stroke from exposure to high heat. Treatment includes evaporative cooling, rehydration, and supportive treatment according to organ involvement.

Hypothermia

Hypothermia occurs with exposure to low temperatures that cause the core body temperature to fall below 95 °F (35 °C). Hypothermia may be associated with immersion in cold water, exposure to cold temperature, metabolic disorders (hypothyroidism, hypoglycemia, hypoadrenalism), or CNS abnormalities (head trauma, Wernicke disease). Many patients with hypothermia are intoxicated with alcohol or drugs.

Symptoms of hypothermia include pallor, cold skin, drowsiness, alterations in mental status, confusion, and severe shivering. The patient can progress to shock, coma, dysrhythmias (T-wave inversion and prolongation of PR, QRS, and QT) including atrial fibrillation and AV block, and cardiac arrest.

Diagnosis requires low-reading thermometers to verify temperature.

Treatment includes:

- Passive rewarming if cardiac status stable
- Active rewarming (external) with immersion in warm water or heating blankets at 40 °C, radiant heat
- Active rewarming (internal) with warm humidified oxygen or air inhalation, heated IV fluids, and internal (bladder, peritoneal pleural, GI) lavage
- Warming with extracorporeal circuit, such as arteriovenous or venovenous shunt that warms the blood
- Supportive treatment as indicated

Acid Base Imbalances

Invasive Blood Gas Monitoring

Invasive blood gas monitoring options include the following:

- **Arterial blood gas (ABG)** is the most informative measurement of blood gas status. If an arterial catheter is in place, it is easily obtained by aspirating 1-2 mL of blood.
- **Venous blood gas (VBG)** is easier to obtain if an arterial catheter is not in place. In order to compare the values in the VBG with an ABG, make the following calculations:
    - Add 0.05 to the pH of the VBG.
    - Subtract 5-10 mmHg from the PCO_2 of the VBG.
- **Capillary Blood Gas (CBG)** can be obtained with a heel stick, without a venous or arterial line, but the values obtained in a CBG are the least accurate and are rarely useful. This is used most often in neonates.

COMPONENTS OF A BLOOD GAS READING
The following are components of a blood gas reading:

- **pH** measures the circulating acid and base levels. Neutral pH for humans is 7.4. A value below 7.35 indicates acidosis and a value greater than 7.45 indicates alkalosis.
- **pCO$_2$** is the partial pressure of carbon dioxide and it determines the respiratory component of pH. An elevated pCO$_2$ lowers the pH. A low pCO$_2$ raises the pH. The pCO$_2$ value is dependent on adequate pulmonary ventilation and respiration. Changes in respiratory status quickly alter this value. Normal value range for pCO$_2$ is 35-45 mmHg.
- **pO$_2$** is the partial pressure of oxygen, which indicates how well the individual is transporting oxygen from the lungs into the bloodstream. Normal value is 75-100 mmHg.
- **HCO$_3^-$** is bicarbonate, the metabolic component of pH. This value may slowly change in response to abnormal pH, or a disease process may cause an elevation or depression. Low values decrease the pH and high values raise the pH. Normal value for bicarbonate is 22-26 mEq/L.

METABOLIC AND RESPIRATORY ACIDOSIS
PATHOPHYSIOLOGY
- Metabolic acidosis
    - Increase in fixed acid and inability to excrete acid, or loss of base, with compensatory increase of CO$_2$ excretion by lungs
- Respiratory acidosis
    - Hypoventilation and CO$_2$ retention with renal compensatory retention of bicarbonate (HCO$_3$) and increased excretion of hydrogen

LABORATORY
- Metabolic acidosis
    - Decreased serum pH (<7.35) and PCO$_2$ normal if uncompensated and decreased if compensated
    - Decreased HCO$_3$
- Respiratory acidosis
    - Decreased serum pH (< 7.35) and increased PCO$_2$
    - Increased HCO$_3$ if compensated and normal if uncompensated

CAUSES
- Metabolic acidosis
    - DKA, lactic acidosis, diarrhea, starvation, renal failure, shock, renal tubular acidosis, starvation
- Respiratory acidosis
    - COPD, overdose of sedative or barbiturate (leading to hypoventilation), obesity, severe pneumonia/atelectasis, muscle weakness (Guillain-Barré), mechanical hypoventilation

Symptoms

- Metabolic acidosis
  - Neuro/muscular: Drowsiness, confusion, headache, coma
  - Cardiac: Decreased BP, arrhythmias, flushed skin
  - GI: Nausea, vomiting, abdominal pain, diarrhea
  - Respiratory: Deep inspired tachypnea
- Respiratory acidosis
  - Neuro/muscular: Drowsiness, dizziness, headache, coma, disorientation, seizures
  - Cardiac: Flushed skin, VF, ↓BP
  - GI: Absent
  - Respiratory: Hypoventilation with hypoxia

Metabolic and Respiratory Alkalosis

Pathophysiology

- Metabolic alkalosis
  - Decreased strong acid or increased base with possible compensatory CO_2 retention by lungs
- Respiratory alkalosis
  - Hyperventilation and increased excretion of CO_2 with compensatory HCO_3 excretion by kidneys

Laboratory

- Metabolic alkalosis
  - Increased serum pH (>7.45)
  - PCO_2 normal if uncompensated and increased if compensated
  - Increased HCO_3
- Respiratory alkalosis
  - Increased serum pH (>7.45)
  - Decreased PCO_2
  - HCO_3 normal if uncompensated and decreased if compensated

Causes

- Metabolic alkalosis
  - Excessive vomiting, gastric suctioning, diuretics, potassium deficit, excessive mineralocorticoids and $NaHCO_3$ intake
- Respiratory alkalosis
  - Hyperventilation associated with hypoxia, pulmonary embolus, exercise, anxiety, pain, and fever
  - Encephalopathy, septicemia, brain injury, salicylate overdose, and mechanical hyperventilation

SYMPTOMS

- Metabolic alkalosis
    - Neuromuscular: Dizziness, confusion, nervousness, anxiety, tremors, muscle cramping, tetany, tingling, seizures
    - Cardiac: Tachycardia and arrhythmias
    - GI: Nausea, vomiting, anorexia
    - Respiratory: Compensatory hypoventilation
- Respiratory alkalosis
    - Neuro/muscular: Light-headedness, confusion, lethargy
    - Cardiac: Tachycardia and arrhythmias
    - GI: Epigastric pain, nausea, and vomiting
    - Respiratory: Hyperventilation

Electrolyte Imbalances

SODIUM

Sodium (**Na**) regulates fluid volume, osmolality, acid-base balance, and activity in the muscles, nerves, and myocardium. It is the primary **cation** (positive ion) in extracellular fluid (ECF), necessary to maintain ECF levels that are needed for tissue perfusion:

- Normal range: 135-145 mEq/L
- Hyponatremia: <135 mEq/L
- Hypernatremia: >145 mEq/L

Hyponatremia may result from inadequate sodium intake, excess sodium loss through diarrhea, vomiting, or NG suctioning, or illness, such as severe burns, fever, SIADH, and ketoacidosis.

- **Symptoms**: Irritability to lethargy and alterations in consciousness, cerebral edema with seizures and coma, dyspnea to respiratory failure.
- **Treatment**: Identify and treat underlying cause and provide Na replacement.

Hypernatremia may result from renal disease, diabetes insipidus, and fluid depletion.

- **Symptoms**: Irritability to lethargy to confusion to coma; seizures; flushing; muscle weakness and spasms; thirst.
- **Treatment**: Identify and treat underlying cause, monitor Na levels carefully, and give IV fluid replacement.

POTASSIUM

Potassium (**K**) is the primary **electrolyte** in intracellular fluid (ICF) with about 98% inside cells and only 2% in ECF, although this small amount is important for neuromuscular activity. Potassium influences activity of the skeletal and cardiac muscles. Its level is dependent upon adequate renal functioning because 80% is excreted through the kidneys and 20% through the bowels and sweat:

- Normal range: 3.5-5.5 mEq/L
- Hypokalemia: <3.5 mEq/L. Critical value: <2.5 mEq/L
- Hyperkalemia: >5.5 mEq/L. Critical value: >6.5 mEq/L

A healthy NPO patient will need about 40 mEq of K per day to maintain serum K levels. (expect alterations in renal disease and other disease processes).

Hypokalemia is caused by loss of potassium through diarrhea, vomiting, gastric suction, and diuresis, alkalosis, decreased intake with starvation, and nephritis.

- **Symptoms**: Lethargy and weakness; nausea and vomiting; paresthesia and tetany; muscle cramps with hyporeflexia; hypotension; dysrhythmias with EKG changes: PVCs or flattened T-waves.
- **Treatment**: Treatment involves identifying and treating the underlying cause and replacing K. When possible, oral replacement is preferable to IV, as it allows slower adjustment of K levels. When given IV, K should be given no faster than 20 mEq/hour via central line if possible. If given peripherally, 10 mEq/hour is preferable for patient comfort.

Hyperkalemia is caused by renal disease, adrenal insufficiency, metabolic acidosis, severe dehydration, burns, hemolysis, and trauma. It rarely occurs without renal disease but may be induced by treatment (such as NSAIDs and potassium-sparing diuretics). Untreated renal failure results in reduced excretion. Those with Addison's disease and deficient adrenal hormones suffer sodium loss that results in potassium retention.

- **Symptoms**: The primary symptoms relate to the effect on the cardiac muscle: ventricular arrhythmias with increasing changes in EKG lead to cardiac and respiratory arrest, weakness with ascending paralysis and hyperreflexia, diarrhea, and increasing confusion.
- **Treatment**: Treatment includes identifying the underlying cause and discontinuing sources of increased K. Calcium gluconate to decrease cardiac effects. Sodium bicarbonate shifts K into the cells temporarily. Insulin and hypertonic dextrose shift K into the cells temporarily. Cation exchange resin (Kayexalate®) to decrease K. Peritoneal dialysis or hemodialysis to remove excess K.

Note: When a tourniquet is on, a patient opening and closing their hand can lead to falsely elevated K levels.

Calcium

More than 99% of calcium (**Ca**) is in the skeletal system with 1% in serum, but it is important for transmitting nerve impulses and regulating muscle contraction and relaxation, including the myocardium. Calcium activates enzymes that stimulate chemical reactions and has a role in coagulation of blood:

- Normal range: 8.2 to 10.2 mg/dL
- Hypocalcemia: <8.2. Critical value: <7 mg/dL
- Hypercalcemia: >10.2 mg/dL. Critical value: >12 mg/dL

Hypercalcemia may be caused by acidosis, kidney disease, hyperparathyroidism, prolonged immobilization, and malignancies. Crisis carries a 50% mortality rate.

- **Symptoms**: Increasing muscle weakness with hypotonicity; anorexia; nausea and vomiting; constipation; bradycardia and cardiac arrest.
- **Treatment**: Identify and treat underlying cause, loop diuretics, IV fluids, phosphate.

Hypocalcemia may be caused by a damage to the parathyroid resulting in hypoparathyroidism (directly decreasing calcium production), vitamin D resistance or inadequacy, or liver/kidney disease.

- **Symptoms**: Muscle cramping or spasms; seizures; numbness or tingling of the feet, hands, or lips; tetany if severe.
- **Treatment**: Identify and treat underlying cause, replace calcium by administering IV calcium gluconate in acute circumstances or increasing oral Vitamin D and calcium in chronic cases.

Phosphorus

Phosphorus, or phosphate, (PO_4) is necessary for neuromuscular and red blood cell function, the maintenance of acid-base balance, and provides structure for teeth and bones. About 85% is in the bones, 14% in soft tissue, and <1% in ECF.

- Normal range: 2.4-4.5 mEq/L
- Hypophosphatemia: <2.4 mEq/L
- Hyperphosphatemia: >4.5 mEq/L

Hypophosphatemia occurs with severe protein-calorie malnutrition, excess antacids with magnesium, calcium, or aluminum, hyperventilation, severe burns, and diabetic ketoacidosis.

- **Symptoms**: Irritability, tremors, seizures to coma; hemolytic anemia; decreased myocardial function; respiratory failure.
- **Treatment**: Identify and treat underlying cause and replace phosphorus.

Hyperphosphatemia occurs with renal failure, hypoparathyroidism, excessive intake, and neoplastic disease, diabetic ketoacidosis, muscle necrosis, and chemotherapy.

- **Symptoms**: Tachycardia; muscle cramping; hyperreflexia and tetany; nausea and diarrhea.
- **Treatment**: Identify and treat underlying cause, correct hypocalcemia, and provide antacids and dialysis.

Magnesium

Magnesium (**Mg**) is the second most common intracellular electrolyte (after potassium) and activates many intracellular enzyme systems. Mg is important for carbohydrate and protein metabolism, neuromuscular function, and cardiovascular function, producing vasodilation and directly affecting the peripheral arterial system:

- Normal range: 1.7-2.2 mg/dL
- Hypomagnesemia critical value: <1.2 mg/dL
- Hypermagnesemia critical value: >4.9 mg/dL

Hypomagnesemia occurs with chronic diarrhea, chronic renal disease, chronic pancreatitis, excess diuretic or laxative use, hyperthyroidism, hypoparathyroidism, severe burns, and diaphoresis.

- **Symptoms**: Neuromuscular excitability or tetany; confusion, headaches, dizziness; seizure and coma; tachycardia with ventricular arrhythmias; respiratory depression.
- **Treatment**: Identify and treat underlying cause, provide magnesium replacement. IV magnesium is a vasodilator, 2 g over 60 mins.

Hypermagnesemia occurs with renal failure or inadequate renal function, diabetic ketoacidosis, hypothyroidism, and Addison's disease.

- **Symptoms**: Muscle weakness, seizures, and dysphagia with decreased gag reflex; tachycardia with hypotension.
- **Treatment**: Identify and treat underlying cause, IV hydration with calcium, and dialysis.

> **Review Video: Fluid and Electrolytes**
> Visit mometrix.com/academy and enter code: 384389

Infection Control

NOSOCOMIAL INFECTIONS

Nosocomial infections are those that are healthcare-associated or hospital-acquired. The following is a list of common nosocomial infections.

- *Enterococci* infections include urinary infections, bacteremia, endocarditis as well as infections in wounds and the abdominal and pelvic areas.
- *Enterobacteriaceae* cause about half of the urinary tract infections and a quarter of the postoperative infections.
- *Escherichia coli* primarily causes urinary tract infections (especially related to catheters), diarrhea, and neonatal meningitis but it can also lead to pneumonia, and bacteremia (usually secondary to urinary infection).
- Group B β-hemolytic *Streptococci* (GBS) has increasingly been a cause of infections in neonatal units, causing pneumonia, meningitis, and sepsis. GBS infections may occur as wound infections after Caesarean sections, especially in those immunocompromised.
- *Staphylococcus aureus* is a major cause of nosocomial post-operative infections, both localized and systemic, and from indwelling tubes and devices.
- Methicillin-resistant *Staphylococcus aureus (MRSA)* is a common cause of surgical infections.
- *Clostridium difficile* causes more nosocomial diarrhea cases than any other microorganism.
- *Candida*, a yeast fungal pathogen, can overgrow and lead to mucocutaneous or cutaneous lesions and sepsis.
- *Aspergillus* spp., filamentous fungi, produce spores that become airborne and can invade the respiratory tract, causing pneumonia.

CATHETER-RELATED INFECTIONS

Intravenous catheter-related infections are a significant cause of morbidity and mortality in the hospital setting. Usually, these infections are due to *Staphylococcus aureus, enterococcus*, or fungal infection such as *Candida*. These infections are important because they may progress and eventually lead to bacteremia, infective endocarditis, septic pulmonary emboli, septic shock, osteomyelitis, or superficial thrombophlebitis. Therefore, vigilance should be maintained to prevent these infections. The patient may exhibit fevers, chills, and discomfort around the catheter site. The site itself may show purulence or erythema. The subclavian vein is the preferred intravenous site and the femoral is the least-preferred site due to high infection rates. Infections are diagnosed with blood cultures and catheter tip cultures. Initial treatment includes removal of the catheter and antibiotic treatment. Antibiotics should be empiric at first, then directed toward culture results. Treatment duration should be 2 weeks at first, but 4-6 weeks if there is a complicated infection.

INFECTION CONTROL MEASURES

Standard infection control measures are designed to prevent transmission of microbial substances between patients and/or medical providers. These measures are indicated for everyone and include frequent handwashing, gloves whenever bodily fluids are involved, and face shields and gowns when splashes are anticipated. For more advanced control with tuberculosis, SARS, vesicular rash disorders (such as VZV), and most recently COVID-19, **airborne precautions** should be instituted to prevent the spread of tiny droplets that can remain suspended in the air for days and travel throughout a hospital environment. Therefore, negative pressure rooms are essential, and providers and patients should wear high-efficiency N95 masks and be fitted in advance. For disorders such as influenza or other infections spread by droplets (spread by cough or sneeze) basic surgical masks should be worn (**droplet precautions**). For **contact precautions** in the setting of fecally-transmitted infection or vesicular rash diseases, gowns/gloves should be used and contact limited. White coats are not a substitute for proper gowning. In the case of a *Clostridium difficile* infection, contact precautions should be used in addition to washing hands with soap and water (rather than alcohol-based hand sanitizer) after patient contact.

INFECTION CONTROL PLAN

The purpose of an infection control/surveillance plan should be clearly outlined and may be multifaceted, including the following elements:

- **Decreasing rates of infection**: The primary purpose of a surveillance plan is to identify a means to decrease nosocomial infections, including a notification system and laboratory surveillance.
- **Evaluating infection control measures**: Surveillance can evaluate effectiveness of infection control measures. (Surgical checklists, handwashing, housekeeping, ventilation).
- **Establishing endemic threshold rates**: Establishing threshold rates can help to enact control measures to reduce rates.
- **Identifying outbreaks**: About 5-10% of infections occur in outbreaks, and comparing data with established endemic threshold rates can help to identify these outbreaks if analysis is done in a regular and timely manner.
- **Achieving staff compliance**: Objective evidence may convince staff to cooperate with infection control measures.
- **Meeting accreditation standards**: Some accreditation agencies require reports of infection rates.
- **Providing defense for malpractice suits**: Providing evidence that a facility is proactive in combating infections can decrease liability.
- **Comparing infection rates with other facilities**: Comparing data helps focus attention and resources.

PROTOCOL FOR NEEDLESTICK INJURY AND POSTEXPOSURE PROPHYLAXIS

If the healthcare provider experiences a **needlestick injury**, the individual's initial response should be to irrigate the wound with soap and water. As soon as possible, the incident must be reported to a supervisor and steps taken according to established protocol. This may include testing and/or prophylaxis, depending on the patient's health history. In some cases, the patient may also be tested for communicable diseases, such as HIV, in order to determine the risk to the healthcare provider. PEP (post-exposure prophylaxis) is available for exposure to HIV (human immunodeficiency virus) and hepatitis B virus (hepatis B immune globulin). However, no PEP is available for HCV (hepatitis C virus) although the CDC does provide a plan for management. PEP should be initiated within 72 hours of exposure. All testing and treatments associated with the needlestick injury must be provided free of cost at a hospital or medical facility.

Infectious Diseases

VIRAL INFECTIONS

HERPES SIMPLEX VIRUS INFECTIONS

There are 2 types of the herpes simplex virus (HSV), human herpesvirus 1 and 2. **HSV-1** usually causes a **gingivostomatitis** (often referred to as "cold sores" or "fever blisters") and is transmitted through **close contact**. HSV-2 usually causes painful **genital lesions** through **sexual contact**. Either may be found in other areas of the body.

- **Incubation** period is around 2-12 days.
- The primary infection is usually more severe (causes systemic **symptoms**) than the reactivated infection, but it may be asymptomatic. After the primary infection, the virus remains dormant in the nerve ganglia, and can be reactivated especially during times of stress, illness, immunosuppression, or sun exposure. While patients are most contagious during times of active lesions, the disease may be spread while asymptomatic. The frequency of the outbreaks usually decreases over time.
- HSV **lesions** are grouped vesicles with an erythematous base. They are usually painful, and a prodrome of tingling, pain, or burning sensations may be felt hours to a couple days before the eruption. Lesions last for approximately 2-3 weeks in primary infection (up to 4 weeks with genital HSV), and 1-2 weeks in recurrent infections.
- HSV is **diagnosed** clinically and confirmed with a + culture, PCR test, or HSV antibody tests (HSV-1 or HSV-2: IgM= active or recent infection; IgG= previous infection).
- Symptomatic **treatment**, proper wound care, and antivirals (acyclovir, valacyclovir, or famciclovir) may be given.
- **Complications** include perinatal infection, keratitis, herpetic whitlow, herpes gladiatorum, secondary infections, and encephalitis.

EPSTEIN-BARR INFECTION

Epstein-Barr virus (EBV) is a **herpesvirus** (human herpesvirus 4) and is responsible for causing **infectious mononucleosis**. After the initial infection, it remains latent in B cells and epithelial cells. It has been linked to certain epithelial and lymphatic neoplasms (e.g., nasopharyngeal carcinoma, Burkitt lymphoma, Hodgkin lymphoma).

- EBV is **transmitted** through **body fluids** like saliva, so it is sometimes referred to as the kissing disease. It is most common in teenagers and college-age young adults
- **Incubation** period is typically 30-50 days.
- **Symptoms** of EBV infection range from being asymptomatic to swollen painful lymph nodes, pharyngitis (can mimic strep pharyngitis), extreme fatigue, fever, and possibly hepatosplenomegaly. The WBC count is elevated (~10,000-20,000 cells/mL) with 10-30% atypical lymphocytes in the differential.
- Confirm **diagnosis** with a Mono Spot test or EBV antibody serology tests.

- **Treatment** is supportive, and antibiotics are not helpful in treating this viral infection. Therefore, avoid unnecessary antibiotics in those with EBV, especially since administration of ampicillin or amoxicillin is often associated with a pruritic, maculopapular rash. Analgesics, warm salt water gargles, increased fluid intake, and rest will help to relieve some of the symptoms. Symptoms may last for several weeks and fatigue may last even longer. Patients should avoid contact sports for up to 2 months.
- **Complications** include hepatitis, cytopenias (e.g., thrombocytopenia), Guillain Barré syndrome, and splenic rupture.

Measles, Mumps, and Rubella

Measles (rubeola) virus is highly contagious, is spread through **respiratory secretions** (incubation is 7-14 days), and peaks in late winter to spring. It causes a prodrome of high fever (4-7 days), cough, congestion, conjunctivitis; then Koplik spots (pathognomonic), and finally a maculopapular rash (spreads cephalocaudally). Report suspected cases immediately to the health dept. **Diagnose** with a + IgM antibody test (collected after 3 days of rash), viral culture, or PCR. **Treatment** is supportive.

Mumps (parotitis) is a viral infection that is spread via **saliva** (incubation is 12-24 days), and often occurs during winter and spring. It causes painful swelling of the salivary glands (parotid). Report to health dept. Supportive **treatment**. Complications include orchitis (infertility), pancreatitis, and meningitis.

Rubella (German measles) is a virus that spreads via **respiratory droplets** (incubation is 2-3 weeks), and peaks in the spring. There is a mild prodrome (fever, aches, sore throat, conjunctivitis, swollen nodes [esp. suboccipital, postauricular, & posterior cervical]), then a maculopapular rash (face 1st then down). Report to health dept. Confirm with rubella antibodies IgM or IgG. Symptomatic care.

Influenza

Influenza is a highly contagious viral infection that affects the entire **respiratory system** from the nose to the lungs. There are 3 types of **influenza virus**: **A** (causes epidemics), **B** (only in humans), and **C**. Types A and B are seen most often and are the strains that the annual flu vaccine is most effective against; and type C is not as common and much less severe.

- Prevention is key and annual, age-appropriate influenza **vaccines** should be given to those ≥6 months; 2 vaccines are required in first-time vaccine patients if 6 mo. through 8-year-olds (separated by 28 days).
- **Incubation** period is 1-4 days and it is spread via respiratory droplets.
- Though **symptoms** can be very similar, the flu and the common cold differ in that the flu has a very sudden onset. Symptoms of influenza include a high fever (may last up to 5 days), headache, myalgias, dry cough, rhinorrhea, and fatigue. There may also be vomiting and diarrhea, although children are more prone to this.
- Clinical judgement, community patterns, and rapid influenza tests (high specificity, but lower sensitivity) aid in **diagnosis**, but RT-PCR or viral culture definitively confirm the diagnosis; pulse oximetry and CXR as needed for pulmonary issues.

- Antibiotic **treatment** is not effective unless there is a secondary bacterial infection (e.g., pneumonia). Look for signs of secondary infections (e.g., dyspnea, cyanosis, fever that goes away and returns, confusion/lethargy). Supportive treatment with rest, fluids, and analgesics. Antivirals should be considered in those who are at high risk (<5 years old, elderly, pregnant, chronic conditions). These are most effective if initiated within 24-48 hours of symptom onset. The neuraminidase inhibitors (oseltamivir, zanamivir) treat type A, type B, and avian H5N1. There is extensive resistance to the adamantanes (amantadine, rimantadine) so they are rarely used.
- **Complications** include pneumonia, ARDS, and death.

CORONAVIRUS

A coronavirus is a common virus that causes cold-like symptoms, including a cough, runny nose, sore throat, and congestion. Most cases of coronavirus are not dangerous and are often given little attention or go entirely unnoticed. However, specific coronavirus strains have led to two worldwide pandemics. The first, **Severe Acute Respiratory Syndrome (SARS)**, appeared in China in 2002 and quickly spread worldwide. Presenting symptoms of SARS were fever, cough, dyspnea, and general malaise. It was extremely virulent, spreading easily from person to person through close contact by way of contaminated droplets produced by coughing or sneezing. SARS was also very deadly, with a case fatality rate of nearly 10%. High rates of infection occurred in health care workers and others in contact with infected patients, so prompt diagnosis and proper isolation were essential. By 2004, there were no longer any documented active cases of SARS.

The most recent coronavirus outbreak was the **COVID-19** strain, which first appeared in December of 2019, in the Chinese city of Wuhan, and quickly became a global pandemic. Presentation of COVID-19 was similar to that of SARS, with the notable additional symptom of acute loss of taste/smell as a unique identifier. Much is still unknown about this strain, including exact transmission methods (though droplet transmission is suspected), effective treatment protocols, and long-term effects.

Precautions to take when treating patients with pandemic coronavirus include the following:

- Contact and droplet precautions, including eye protection and appropriate personal protection equipment.
- Airborne precautions (recommended by the CDC), especially with aerosol-producing procedures (ventilators, nebulizers, intubation).
- Immediate notification of public health authorities and institution of contact tracing.
- Activity restrictions of exposed health care workers planned in coordination with public health officials.

CYTOMEGALOVIRUS

Cytomegalovirus (CMV) is a herpes virus, occurring in most people by the time they are adults.

- **Transmission** can occur through secretions during personal contact and from mother to baby before, during or after birth.
- Most cases have no **symptoms**, although a few infants will have fetal damage, such as jaundice, hepatitis, brain damage, or growth retardation.
- **Treatment** for those with severe infections is with ganciclovir, an antiviral drug.

Respiratory Syncytial Virus

Respiratory syncytial virus (RSV) is a virus that infects the respiratory tract, causing symptoms of nasal congestion, cough, sore throat, and headache. Severe cases can lead to high fever, breathing difficulties, severe cough, and cyanosis.

- Respiratory syncytial virus may **manifest** as a cold in adults and older children; however, there are some children who are more at risk of developing complications.
- **Transmission** is through contact with droplets from an infected person's nose or throat, generally through coughing and sneezing.
- Infants born prematurely, children with chronic lung disease, children with cystic fibrosis, and children who are in an immunocompromised state because of surgery or illness are at **high risk** of breathing difficulties, poor oxygenation, and even death from RSV.

Bacterial Infections

Diphtheria

Diphtheria, caused by ***Corynebacterium diphtheriae***, is most prevalent in fall and winter.

- The **incubation** period is 2-7 days, possibly longer, and transmission is through direct contact with nasal, eye, and oral secretions.
- The **symptoms** are slight fever, nasal discharge, sore throat, feeling unwell, poor appetite, and swelling of the airway.
- If the disease is severe, death can result. The patient requires isolation, bed rest, fluids, antibiotics, medication for fever, and an antitoxin. The patient may also require oxygen therapy and tracheostomy if the airway is obstructed.

Tetanus

Tetanus, caused by ***Clostridium tetani***, occurs all over the world. The spores formed by the bacillus are present in soil, dust, and the GI tracts of animals and humans.

- The **incubation** period is 3-21 days.
- **Symptoms** start with headache, irritability, jaw muscle spasms, and inability to open the mouth. This is followed by severe back muscle spasms, seizures, incontinence, and fever.
- **Treatment** requires human tetanus immune globulin, penicillin G, Valium, and placement on a ventilator. The environment should be kept quiet because the spasms are initiated by stimuli.

Fungal Infections

Cryptococcosis

Cryptococcosis is an infection resulting from inhaling the **fungus** *Cryptococcus neoformans,* which is found worldwide in soil (can be associated with bird droppings), or *Cryptococcus gattii,* which is associated with certain trees in the Northwest.

- Cryptococcosis is most often due to *C. neoformans*. It is often found among those with compromised immune systems and is an **AIDS-defining opportunistic infection**.
- Healthy patients may be asymptomatic and the only finding may be pulmonary lesions on CXR that resolve spontaneously. The fungus can disseminate and cause meningitis, encephalitis, cutaneous lesions, and affect long bones and other tissues. **Symptoms** are based on the area of involvement. Patients may experience cough, pleuritic chest pain, weight loss, and fever if there is pulmonary involvement; headache, double vision, light sensitivity, N/V, and confusion if CNS involvement; cutaneous lesions (papules, pustules, nodules, ulcers) if the skin is involved.
- **Diagnosis** includes microscopic analysis, culture (gold standard), or an antigen test (highly sensitive; good for detecting early infection) for *Cryptococcus* using CSF, tissue, sputum, blood, or urine. Check CSF by India ink (limited sensitivity) or culture so meningitis can be ruled out. Confirm that no mass lesion is present by CT or MRI before LP is performed.
- Mild cases may only require monitoring to ensure that the infection does not spread. In more advanced cases, the infection is treated with different antifungal medications (e.g., fluconazole for pulmonary infections, amphotericin B ± flucytosine for meningitis). The patient should also be monitored for CNS infection and medication side effects. AIDS patients may need lifelong antifungals.
- **Complications** include cryptococcal meningitis, neural deficits, optic nerve damage, and hydrocephalus.

Histoplasmosis

Histoplasmosis is an infection caused by inhalation of **spores** from the fungus *Histoplasma capsulatum* that is found in soil and is associated with bird and bat droppings (e.g., chicken coops, caves).

- Healthy patients are usually asymptomatic and those with symptoms are typically immunocompromised or those who've had a heavy exposure to spores. The primary **pulmonary infection** occurs 3-17 days after exposure and can present with flu-like symptoms. It is typically self-limited but may become chronic. Histoplasmosis can also spread through the **blood** and can cause progressive disseminated disease in the immunocompromised (high mortality rate); this is an **AIDS-defining illness**.
- **Diagnose** through antigen tests (urine, serum), histopathology, or cultures; order a CXR. Mild and even moderate acute pulmonary histoplasmosis may resolve on its own.
- If needed, **treat** mild to moderate infections with itraconazole and severe illness with amphotericin B.

Pneumocystis

Pneumocystis jiroveci is a **fungus** (previously known as *Pneumocystis* carinii) that causes **pneumonia** (PJP, previously PCP) in the immunocompromised. Most people have been exposed to this by the age of 3 or 4.

- **Symptoms** of PJP include a dry nonproductive cough, fever, dyspnea, and weight loss.
- CXR may show diffuse bilateral infiltrates or it may be normal; and pulse oximetry may be low, especially on exertion. **Diagnosis** is confirmed with sputum histopathology using sputum induction or bronchoalveolar lavage.
- **Treat** immediately with TMP-SMX (trimethoprim/sulfamethoxazole) for 21 days if HIV + and for 14 days in other cases. Steroids may be added for HIV patients with severe PJP. HIV/AIDS patients with CD4 counts <200/μL should receive PJP prophylaxis with TMP-SMX. Dapsone and pentamidine are alternatives.
- **Complications** include ARDS and death.

Candidal Infections

Candida is a type of yeast that may cause a variety of infections:

- **Oral thrush** is commonly seen in diabetic patients and those who are immunosuppressed (HIV or underlying neoplasm). Patients often complain of burning on the tongue or in the mouth, associated with "curd-like" white patches that can be scraped away leaving reddish tissue underneath. Diagnosis is with KOH prep. Treatment is with oral or topical antifungals, including nystatin (swish and swallow or troches).
- **Candida esophagitis** also occurs in the immunosuppressed population, and patients may complain of dysphasia, odynophagia, and chest pain. This is diagnosed on EGD and may be treated with oral or IV antifungals (ketoconazole).
- **Candidal intertrigo**, or diaper rash, presents with beefy-red lesions at skin fold areas as well as satellite lesions. Treatment is with topical antifungals.
- **Candidemia** is diagnosed with fungal blood cultures and may lead to osteomyelitis, endocarditis, and other complications. Treatment is with IV antifungals.

Ringworm

Ringworm is caused by an infection from the ***Tinea* fungus**, which produces patches on the skin that have normal centers, giving the appearance of a ring.

- The fungus can cause hair loss and patches of scaly skin that may develop blisters that ooze or crust.
- It is **transmitted** by touching the affected skin or through objects that have touched the affected skin.
- Ringworm may be **diagnosed** by viewing the skin section under a Wood's lamp. Skin cultures may also be taken for examination to identify the fungus. A potassium hydroxide (KOH) exam involves scraping the affected skin and placing the skin sample in KOH to test for the presence of the fungus.

Vector-Borne and Parasitic Infections

Malaria

Malaria is a **blood-borne disease** caused by a **parasite** from the genus *Plasmodium and* found in tropical areas. There are 4 known to cause disease in humans (*P. malariae, P. vivax, P. ovale,* and *P. falciparum*). These protozoa are transmitted by the **female *Anopheles* mosquito**. They travel to the **liver** where they multiply, are released, and then infect the RBCs, where they continue to multiply.

Incubation time can be as little as 9 days or as much as multiple years depending on the species of the infecting parasite.

- **Signs and symptoms** include headache, high fever with shaking chills and sweating (rigors; occurs when merozoites, an immature form of the parasite, are released from RBCs), jaundice, anemia, and hepatosplenomegaly. Take a thorough history including recent travel.
- **Diagnose** with 3 thin and thick blood smears (gold standard) stained with Giemsa (preferred) and obtained 12-24 hours apart. Labs typically show elevated LDH, thrombocytopenia, and atypical lymphocytes. Rapid antigen tests are also available as well as PCR.
- **Treat** with chloroquine. If travelling, chemoprophylaxis depends on the area of travel due to species and resistance patterns, and may include chloroquine, primaquine, mefloquine, Malarone®, or doxycycline. Report infections to your local or state health department.
- **Complications** include severe anemia and hemolysis, organ failure (liver, spleen, kidneys), cerebral malaria, ARDS, and death.

LYME DISEASE

Lyme disease occurs from a bite from a **deer tick** (blacklegged tick) infected with the **spirochete bacterium** *Borrelia burgdorferi*. It is the most common tick-borne disease in the U.S. and is more prevalent in heavily wooded areas. Adult ticks are more active during colder times whereas the nymphs (<2 mm in size) are more active in the warm, spring or summer months. Once the tick bites, it stays attached; however, it takes about 36-48 hours for nymphs and about 48-72 hours for adult ticks before the spirochete is transmitted to the person. **Incubation** period is 3-30 days. There are 3 stages to this disease: early localized, early disseminated, and chronic disseminated.

- At **Stage 1**, 75% have the characteristic expanding red rash (erythema migrans; can be large, ~30cm) which can progress to have central clearing (bull's eye), headache, fever, chills, myalgias, and fatigue.
- **Stage 2** occurs weeks to months after initial infection and involves systemic symptoms (flu-like), neck stiffness, headaches, migrating pain in muscles and joints, rashes, paresthesias, Bell's palsy, confusion, fatigue, myocarditis, and heart palpitations.
- **Stage 3** occurs months to years after initial infection and involves neurologic (e.g., encephalitis) and rheumatologic issues, especially arthritis of large joints (e.g., knee).

DIAGNOSIS AND TREATMENT OF LYME DISEASE

Diagnose Lyme disease using 2-tiered testing: antibodies (IgM, IgG), then Western blot. Antibiotic treatment for localized Lyme disease involves 2-3 weeks of doxycycline, amoxicillin, or cefuroxime axetil is started immediately after diagnosis. IV antibiotics may be needed for severe disease (e.g., IV ceftriaxone). Prevention is key by wearing clothes covering the skin, using tick repellents, showering soon after being outdoors in tick-prone areas, and thoroughly checking for ticks (especially in hard to see areas by using a mirror). The Lyme vaccine is no longer available and previous vaccine recipients are still at risk of contracting the disease as protection decreases over time. Complications are prevalent with untreated Lyme disease and include chronic arthritis, fatigue, chronic musculoskeletal issues, acrodermatitis chronica atrophicans, and memory and concentration issues. Report cases to the local health dept.

Rocky Mountain Spotted Fever

Rocky Mountain spotted fever is a tick-borne illness caused by **Rickettsia rickettsii**. It tends to occur in spring and summer throughout the United States.

- **Incubation** period is about one week.
- **Symptoms** include headache, fever, nausea, vomiting, loss of appetite, muscle pain, and rash on the ankles and wrists.
- **Treatment** requires an antibiotic, usually Vibramycin.

Helminth Infestations

Helminth infestations (worms) include **roundworms** [nematodes: *Ascaris*, hookworms (cause anemia), **filariae** (cause elephantiasis)] and **flatworms** [tapeworms (cause weight loss); **flukes** (intestinal or liver)]. **Pinworms** are a type of roundworm that cause enterobiasis and is the most common helminth infestation. Pinworms are more prevalent in warmer areas of the country and infestations occur more frequently in children. The worms lay eggs within the digestive tract and then travel to the anal area where they are usually found. Pinworms are highly contagious. As a patient itches the anal area where the eggs are located, the eggs cling to the fingers and can easily be transmitted to other people either directly or through food or surfaces. The eggs can survive for 2-3 weeks on inanimate objects.

- Patients may be asymptomatic or have intense anal itching that is usually worse at night and can cause insomnia. Abdominal pain, nausea, and vomiting can also occur.
- **Diagnose** with the "tape test" which involves pressing cellophane tape over the perianal area to pick up eggs or worms and examine under the microscope. Most other helminth infestations can be diagnosed with a stool sample for ova and parasites; filariasis requires a blood smear or antigen test.
- Anthelmintic medications are given in a single dose and repeated in 2 weeks to kill the pinworms and their larvae (mebendazole, albendazole, or pyrantel pamoate). The entire family and close contacts should be treated simultaneously since pinworms are so contagious.

Giardia Lamblia

Giardia lamblia is a **protozoan** that infects water supplies and spreads to children through the fecal-oral route. It is the most common cause of non-bacterial diarrhea in the United States, causing about 20,000 cases of infection each year in all ages.

- Children often become infected after swallowing recreational waters (pools, lakes) while swimming or putting contaminated items into the mouth. *Giardia* live and multiply within the small intestine where cysts develop.
- **Symptoms** occur 7-14 days after ingestion of 1 or more cysts and include diarrhea with greasy floating stools (rarely bloody), stomach cramps, nausea, and flatulence, lasting 2-6 weeks. A chronic infection may develop that can last for months or years.
- **Treatment** includes Furazolidone 5-8 mg/kg/day in 4 doses for 7-10 days or Metronidazole 40 mg/kg/day in 3 doses for 7-10 days. Chronic infections are often very resistant to treatment.

Toxoplasmosis

Toxoplasmosis is an infection caused by the **parasite *Toxoplasma gondii***, which is commonly found in soil. It is widespread and transmitted through cat feces; however, it also may be contracted by eating undercooked meat (especially pork, lamb, or venison) or poorly washed vegetables.

Toxoplasmosis can cause serious disease and can affect various organs; and immunocompromised and pregnant women and their unborn babies are especially likely to have side effects of the disease (the "T" in congenital TORCH infections).

- Healthy patients are usually asymptomatic; however, once infected the parasite can remain latent until the patient becomes immunocompromised and the parasite is reactivated causing **symptoms**. The disease can cause a flu-like illness with fever, myalgias, and lymphadenopathy. More serious effects include retinochoroiditis, brain lesions, and encephalitis. Congenital toxoplasmosis may cause retinochoroiditis, microcephaly, hydrocephalus, intellectual disability, and possibly miscarriage or stillbirth.
- **Diagnose** with serology for *Toxoplasma* antibodies IgM and IgG. Also, PCR may be used to test amniotic fluid, CSF, or tissue.
- **Treat** with pyrimethamine (preferred) plus folinic acid or sulfadiazine plus folinic acid. Pregnant women should avoid high-risk practices like changing the cat litter and should avoid sand boxes.

Psychosocial Pathophysiology

BIPOLAR DISORDER

Bipolar disorder causes severe mood swings between hyperactive states and depression, accompanied by impaired judgment because of distorted thoughts. The hypomanic stage may allow for creativity and good functioning in some people, but it can develop into more severe mania, which may be associated with psychosis and hallucinations with rapid speech and bizarre behavior, and then into periods of profound depression. While most cases are diagnosed in late adolescence, there is increasing evidence that some children present with symptoms earlier; especially at risk are children with a bipolar parent. Bipolar disorder is associated with high rates of suicide, so early diagnosis and treatment is critical.

Symptoms may be relatively mild or involve severe rapid cycling between mania and depression.

Treatment includes both medications (usually given continually) to prevent cycling and control depression and psychosocial therapy, such as cognitive therapy, to help control disordered thought patterns and behavior. Psychiatric referral should be made.

DEPRESSION

Depression is a mood disorder characterized by profound feelings of sadness and withdrawal. It may be acute (such as after a death) or chronic with recurring episodes over a lifetime. The cause appears to be a combination of genetic, biological, and environmental factors. A major depressive episode is a depressed mood, profound and constant sense of hopelessness and despair, or loss of interest in all or almost all activities for a period of at least two weeks. Some drugs may precipitate depression: diuretics, Parkinson's drugs, estrogen, corticosteroids, cimetidine, hydralazine, propranolol, digitalis, and indomethacin. Depression is associated with neurotransmitter dysregulation, especially serotonin and norepinephrine. Major depression can be mild, moderate, or severe.

Symptoms include changes in mood, sadness, loss of interest in usual activities, increased fatigue, changes in appetite and fluctuations in weight, anxiety, and sleep disturbance.

Treatment includes tricyclic antidepressants (TCAS) and SSRIs, but SSRIs have fewer side effects and are less likely to cause death with an overdose. Counselling, undergoing cognitive behavioral therapy, treating underlying cause, and instituting an exercise program may help reduce depression.

ANXIETY AND DEPRESSION DUE TO INTENSIVE CARE STAYS

Anxiety and depression affect over half of patients who are treated in intensive care not only during the stay but also after discharge, especially if care is long-term or if their needs for moderate or high care continue. Additionally, studies have shown that those who suffer depression during and after ICU stays have increased risk of mortality over the next two years. Patients with anxiety may appear restless (thrashing about the bed), have difficulty concentrating, exhibit tachycardia and tachypnea, experience insomnia and feelings of dread, and complain of various ailments, such as stomach ache and headache. Symptoms of depression may overlap (and patients may have both anxiety and depression) and may also include fatigue, insomnia, withdrawal, appetite change, irritability, pessimistic outlooks, feelings of worthlessness, sadness, and suicidal ideation. Brief screening tools for anxiety and depression should be used with all ICU patients and interventions per psychological referral made as needed.

ANXIETY DISORDERS

Anxiety is a human emotion and experience that everyone has at some point during their life. Feelings of uncertainty, helplessness, isolation, alienation, and insecurity can all be experienced during an **anxiety response**. Many times, anxiety occurs without a specific known object or source. It can occur because of the unknown. Anxiety occurs throughout the life cycle, and therefore anxiety disorders can affect people of all ages. Populations that are most commonly affected include women, smokers, people under the age of 45, individuals that are separated or divorced, victims of abuse, and people in the lower socioeconomic groups. An individual can have one single anxiety disorder, experience more than one anxiety disorder, or have other mental health disorders all occurring at the same time.

GENERALIZED ANXIETY DISORDER

Generalized anxiety disorder can be very insidious and occurs when an individual consistently experiences **excessive anxiety and worry**. This anxiety and worry will be present almost every day and lasts for a period of at least six months. The worry and anxiety will be uncontrollable, intrusive, and not related to any medical disease process. It will pertain to real-life events, situations, or circumstances and may occur along with mild depression symptoms. The individual will also experience three or more of the following symptoms: fatigue, inability to concentrate, irritability, insomnia, restlessness, loosing thought processes or going blank, and muscle tension. The continued anxiety and worry will eventually affect daily functioning and cause social and occupational disturbances.

COMORBIDITIES

Individuals with generalized anxiety disorder (GAD) will often have **other mental health disorders**. When a person has more than one psychological disorder occurring at the same time, these disorders are considered to be **comorbid**. Most patients suffering from GAD will have at least one more psychiatric diagnosis. The most common comorbid disorders can include major depressive disorder, social or specific phobias, panic disorder, and dysthymic disorder. It is also common for these individuals to have substance abuse problems, and they may look to alcohol or barbiturates to help control their symptoms of anxiety.

LEVELS OF ANXIETY

There are four main levels of anxiety that were named by Peplau. They are as follows:

1. **Mild anxiety** is associated with normal tensions of everyday life. It can increase awareness and motivate learning and creativity.
2. **Moderate anxiety** occurs when the individual narrows their field of perception and focuses on the immediate problem. This level decreases the perceptual field; however, the person can tend to other tasks if directed.
3. **Severe anxiety** leads to a markedly reduced field of perception and the person focuses only on the details of the problem. All energy is directed at relieving the anxiety and the person can only perform other tasks under significant persuasion.
4. **Panic** is the most extreme level of anxiety and associated with feelings of dread and terror. The individual is unable to perform any other tasks no matter how strongly they are persuaded to do so. This level can be life-threatening with complete disorganization of thought occurring.

PHYSICAL SYMPTOMS

Anxiety produces a very physical response and effects the largest body systems, such as cardiovascular, respiratory, GI, neuromuscular, urinary tract, and skin. Symptoms vary and can increase upon a continuum depending upon the level of anxiety the person is experiencing.

- **Cardiovascular symptoms** can include palpitation, tachycardia, hypertension, feeling faint or actually fainting, hypotension, or bradycardia.
- **Respiratory symptoms** can include tachypnea, shortness of breath, chest pressure, shallow respirations, or choking sensation.
- **GI symptoms** can include revulsion toward food, nausea, diarrhea, and abdominal pain or discomfort.

Even though anxiety occurs psychologically, it can produce extreme **physical responses** from the neuromuscular system, urinary tract, and skin. These symptoms can range from mild to severe depending upon the degree of anxiety the person is experiencing.

- **Neuromuscular symptoms** can include hyperreflexia, being easily startled, eyelid twitching, inability to sleep, shaking, fidgeting, pacing, wobbly legs, or clumsy movements.
- **Urinary tract symptoms** can include increased frequency and sensation of need to urinate.
- **Skin symptoms** can include flushed face, sweaty palms, itching, sensations of being hot and/or cold, pale facial coloring, or diaphoresis.

BEHAVIORAL AND AFFECTIVE RESPONSES

Behavioral and affective symptoms along with a multitude of physical symptoms are observable in anxious patients. The effects of these responses can affect the person experiencing the anxiety along with their relationships with others.

- Some **behavioral responses** can include restlessness and physical tension, hypervigilance, rapid speech, social or relationship withdrawal, decreased coordination, avoidance, or flight.
- **Affective responses** are the patient's emotional reactions and can be described subjectively by the individual. Patients may describe symptoms such as edginess, impatience, tension, nervousness, fear, frustration, jitteriness, or helplessness.

COGNITIVE RESPONSES

Anxiety not only produces physical and emotional symptoms, but it can also greatly affect the individual's intellectual abilities. **Cognitive responses** to anxiety occur in three main categories. These include sensory-perceptual, thought difficulties, and conceptualization. Responses that affect the patient's **sensory-perceptual fields** can include feeling that their mind is unclear or clouded, seeing objects indistinctly, perceiving a surreal environment, increased self-consciousness, or hypervigilance. **Thinking difficulties** can include the inability to remember important information, confusion, inability to focus thoughts or attention, easily distracted, blocking thoughts, difficulty with reasoning, tunnel vision, or loss of objectivity. **Conceptual difficulties** can include the fear of loss of control, inability to cope, potential physical injury, developing a mental disorder, or receiving a negative evaluation. The patient may have cognitive distortion, protruding scary visual images, or uncontrollable repetition of fearful thoughts.

PANIC ATTACKS

Panic attacks are short episodes (peaking in 5-10 minutes) of intense anxiety that can result in a wide variety of **symptoms** that include:

- Dyspnea
- Palpitations
- Hyperventilation
- Nausea and vomiting
- Intense fear or anxiety
- Pain and pressure in the chest
- Dizziness and fainting
- Tremors

Panic attacks may be associated with agoraphobia, depression, or intimate partner violence and abuse (IPVA), so a careful history is important. Typically, patients believe they are dying or having a heart attack and require reassurance and treatment, such as diazepam or lorazepam, in the ED for the acute episode. In severe cases, ASA may be given and EKG done to rule out cardiac abnormalities. Patients should be referred for psychiatric evaluation for ongoing medications such as SSRIs (sertraline, paroxetine, fluoxetine) to prevent recurrence. Panic attacks become chronic panic disorders if they are recurrent, with each attack each followed by at least a month of fear of another attack.

PTSD

Patients that experience a traumatic event may re-experience the trauma through distressing thoughts and recollections of the event. In addition, psychological effects of the trauma may include difficulty sleeping, emotional lability and problems with memory and concentration. Patients may also wish to avoid places or activities that remind them of their trauma. These are all characteristics of **post-traumatic stress disorder (PTSD)** and may cause patients extreme distress and significantly impact their quality of life.

Signs and symptoms: Nightmares, flashbacks, insomnia, symptoms of hyperarousal including irritability and anxiety, avoidance, and negative thoughts and feelings about oneself and others.

Diagnosis: PTSD is diagnosed through psychological assessment and criteria defined in the Diagnostic and Statistical Manual of Mental Disorders, Fifth Edition (DSM-5).

Treatment: Pharmacologic therapy may be utilized to help control the symptoms of PTSD. Non-pharmacologic therapy options include group and individual/family therapy, cognitive behavioral therapy, and anxiety management/relaxation techniques. Hypnosis may also be utilized.

STRESS

RELATIONSHIP BETWEEN STRESS AND DISEASE

Stress causes a number of physical and psychological changes within the body:

- Cortisol levels increase
- Digestion is hindered and the colon stimulated
- Heart rate increases
- Perspiration increases
- Anxiety and depression occur and can result in insomnia, anorexia or weight gain, and suicide
- Immune response decreases, making the person more vulnerable to infections
- Autoimmune reaction may increase, leading to autoimmune diseases

The body's **compensatory mechanisms** try to restore homeostasis. When these mechanisms are overwhelmed, pathophysiological injury to the cells of the body result. When this injury begins to interfere with the function of the organs or systems in the body, symptoms of dysfunction will occur. If the conditions are not corrected, the body changes the structure or function of the affected organs or systems.

ADAPTATION OF CELLS TO STRESS

The most common stressors to cells include the lack of oxygen, presence of toxins or chemicals, and infection. **Cells react to stress** by making the following changes:

- **Hypertrophy**: Cells swell, leading to an overall increase in the size of the affected organ.
- **Atrophy**: Cells shrivel and the overall organ size decreases in size.
- **Hyperplasia**: The cells divide and overgrowth and thickening of the tissue results.
- **Dysplasia**: The cells are changed in appearance as a result of irritation over an extended period of time, sometimes leading to malignancy.
- **Metaplasia**: Cells change type as a result of stress.

If the stress that caused the cells to change continues, the cells become injured and die. When enough cells die, organ and systemic failure occur.

PSYCHOLOGICAL RESPONSE TO STRESS

When stress is encountered, a person **responds** according to the threat perceived to compensate. The threat is evaluated as to the amount of harm or loss that has occurred or is possible. If the stress is benign (such as with marriage), then a challenge is present that demands change. Once the threat or challenge is defined, the person can gather information, resources, and support to make the changes needed to resolve the stress to the greatest degree possible. Immediate psychological response to stress may include shock, anger, fear, or excitement. Over time, people may develop chronic anxiety, depression, flashbacks, thought disturbances, and sleep disturbances. Changes may occur in emotions and thinking, in behavior, or in the person's environment. People may be more able to adapt to stress if they have many varied experiences, a good self-esteem, and a support network to help as needed. A healthy lifestyle and philosophical beliefs, including religion, may give a person more reserve to cope with stress.

IMPACT OF DIFFERENT KINDS OF STRESS

Everyone encounters **stress** in life and it **impacts** each person differently. There are the small daily "hassles," major traumatic events, and the periodic stressful events of marriage, birth, divorce, and death. Compounded stress experienced on a daily basis can impact health status over time. Stressors that occur suddenly are the hardest to overcome and result in the greatest tension. The length of time that a stressor is present affects the impact with long-term, relentless stress, such as that generated by poverty or disability, resulting in disease more often. If there is **ineffective coping**, a person will suffer greater changes resulting in even more stress. The nurse can help patients to recognize those things that induce stress in their lives, find ways to reduce stress when possible, and teach effective coping skills and problem-management.

SUICIDAL IDEATION

Patients may attempt suicide for many reasons, including severe depression, social isolation, situational crisis, bereavement, or psychotic disorder.

Suicidal indications are as follows:

- Depression or dysphoria
- Hostility to others
- Problems with peer relationships, and lack of close friends
- Post-crisis stress (divorce, death in family, graduation, college)
- Withdrawn personality; quiet or lonely appearance or behavior
- Change in behavior (dropping grades, unkempt appearance, change in sleeping patterns)
- A sudden increase in positive mood may indicate patient has a plan
- Co-morbid psychiatric problems (bipolar, schizophrenia)
- Substance abuse

The following are indicators of **high risk for repeated suicide attempt**:

- Violent suicide attempt (knives, gunshots)
- Suicide attempt with low chance of rescue
- Ongoing psychosis or disordered thinking
- Ongoing severe depression and feeling of helplessness
- History of previous suicide attempts
- Lack of social support system

Nursing considerations: Take all suicidal ideations seriously; do not minimize them. Suicidal patients should be watched continuously, given plastic utensils, break-away wall rails/shower heads, no cords/sharp instruments.

SUBSTANCE ABUSE

Substance abuse is the abuse of drugs, medicines, or alcohol that causes mental and physical problems for the abuser and family. Abusers use substances out of boredom, to hide negative self-esteem, to dampen emotional pain, and to cope with daily stress. As the abuse continues, abusers become unable to take care of daily needs and duties. They lack effective coping mechanisms and the ability to make healthy choices. They can't identify and prioritize stress or choose positive behavior to resolve the stress in a healthy way. Some family members may act as codependents because of their desire to feel needed by the abuser, to control the person, and to stay with him or her. The nurse can help the family to confront an individual with their concerns about the person and their proposals for treatment. Family members can enforce consequences if treatment is not sought. Family members may also need counseling to learn new behaviors to stop enabling the abuser to continue substance abuse.

PATHOPHYSIOLOGY OF ADDICTION

Genetic, social, and personality factors may all play a role in the development of **addictive tendencies**. However, the main factor of the development of substance addiction is the pharmacological activation of the **reward system** located in the central nervous system (CNS). This reward systems pathway involves **dopaminergic neurons**. Dopamine is found in the CNS and is one of many neurotransmitters that play a role in an individual's mood. The mesolimbic pathway seems to play a primary role in the reward and motivational process involved with addiction. This pathway begins in the ventral tegmental area of the brain (VTA) and then moves forward into the nucleus accumbens located in the middle forebrain bundle (MFB). Some drugs enhance mesolimbic dopamine activity, therefore producing very potent effects on mood and behavior.

INDICATORS OF SUBSTANCE ABUSE

Many people with substance abuse (alcohol or drugs) are reluctant to disclose this information, but there are a number of **indicators** that are suggestive of substance abuse:

Physical signs include:

- Burns on fingers or lips
- Pupils abnormally dilated or constricted, eyes watery
- Slurring of speech, slow speech
- Lack of coordination, instability of gait, tremors
- Sniffing repeatedly, nasal irritation, persistent cough
- Weight loss
- Dysrhythmias
- Pallor, puffiness of face
- Needle tracks on arms or legs
- Odor of alcohol/marijuana on clothing or breath

Behavioral signs include:

- Labile emotions, including mood swings, agitation, and anger
- Inappropriate, impulsive, or risky behavior
- Lying
- Missing appointments
- Difficulty concentrating, short term memory loss, blackouts
- Insomnia or excessive sleeping; disoriented, confused
- Lack of personal hygiene

ALCOHOL WITHDRAWAL

Chronic abuse of ethanol (alcoholism) can lead to physical dependency. Sudden cessation of drinking, which often happens in the inpatient setting, is associated with **alcohol withdrawal syndrome**. It may be precipitated by trauma or infection and has a high mortality rate, 5-15% with treatment and 35% without treatment.

Signs/Symptoms: Anxiety, tachycardia, headache, diaphoresis, progressing to severe agitation, hallucinations, auditory/tactile disturbances, and psychotic behavior (delirium tremens).

Diagnosis: Physical assessment, blood alcohol levels (on admission).

Treatment includes:

- Medication: IV benzodiazepines to manage symptoms; electrolyte and nutritional replacement, especially magnesium and thiamine.
- Use the CIWA scale to measure symptoms of withdrawal; treat as indicated.
- Provide an environment with minimal sensory stimulus (lower lights, close blinds) & implement fall and seizure precautions.
- Prevention: Screen all patients for alcohol/substance abuse, using CAGE or other assessment tool. Remember to express support and comfort to patient; wait until withdrawal symptoms are subsiding to educate about alcohol use and moderation.

EATING DISORDERS
ANOREXIA NERVOSA

Eating disorders are a profound health risk and can lead to death, especially for adolescent girls, although boys also have eating disorders, often presenting as excessive exercise. Anorexia nervosa is characterized by profound fear of weight gain and severe restriction of food intake, often accompanied by abuse of diuretics and laxatives, which can cause electrolyte imbalances, kidney and bowel disorders, and delay or cessation of menses.

- **Symptoms** include growth retardation, amenorrhea (missing 3 consecutive periods), unexplained and sometimes precipitous weight loss (at least 15% below normal weight), dehydration, loss of appetite, hypoglycemia, hypercholesterolemia, or carotenemia with yellowing of skin, emaciated appearance, osteoporosis, bradycardia, and food obsessions and rituals.
- **Diagnosis** includes complete history, physical, and psychological exam with CBC and chemical panels to rule out other disorders.
- **Treatment** includes volume and electrolyte replacement initially with referral to psychiatric care for long-term management of the disorder and nutritional plans.

BULIMIA NERVOSA

Bulimia nervosa includes binge eating followed by vomiting (at least 2 times monthly for at least 3 months), often along with diuretics, enemas, and laxatives. Some may engage in periods of fasting or excessive exercise rather than vomiting to offset the effects of binging. Gastric acids from purging can damage the throat and teeth. While bulimics may maintain a normal weight, they are at risk for severe electrolyte imbalances that can be life-threatening. Binge eating affects 2% to 5% of females and includes grossly overeating, often resulting in obesity, depression, and shame. Symptoms include hypokalemia, metabolic acidosis, fluctuations of weight, dental caries and loss of enamel, knuckle scars (from contact with teeth while inducing vomiting), parotid and submandibular gland enlargement, and insulin-dependent diabetes. Diagnosis includes complete history, physical, and psychological exam with CBC and chemical panels to rule out other disorders. Treatment includes volume and electrolyte replacement initially with referral to psychiatric care for long-term management of the disorder and nutritional plans, as well as SSRIs, naltrexone, and ondansetron.

Psychosocial Procedures and Interventions

PSYCHIATRIC AND MENTAL HEALTH PROGRAMS

A variety of psychiatric and mental health programs are available and should be evaluated, according to the needs of the individual patient.

- **Inpatient programs** provide a secure environment and comprehensive care, often with psychologists, psychiatrists, occupational therapists, social workers, and other allied health personnel. Programs may be tailored to one specific type of patient (e.g., criminally insane, substance abusers) or to a general population. They may offer short-term or long-term care.
- **Outpatient programs** provide assessment and treatment, such as group therapy, cognitive-behavioral therapy, and family therapy. Programs may be community-based, targeting specific groups of people, such as alcoholics or the homeless.
- **Partial/day hospitalization programs** provide daily inpatient care during prescribed hours (e.g., 8 a.m. to 3 p.m.) as well as outpatient services. The stay is usually short-term (1–2 weeks) and may serve as a transition from inpatient to outpatient care.

NONVIOLENT CRISIS INTERVENTION AND DE-ESCALATION TECHNIQUES

Nonviolent crisis intervention and de-escalation techniques begin with self-awareness because the normal response to aggression is a stress response (freezing, fight/flight, fear). The nurse must control these responses in order to deal with the situation. The nurse should recognize signs of impending conflict (clenched fists, and sudden change in tone of voice or body stance, and change in eye contact). Steps include:

- Maintain social distance (≥12 feet) if possible and stay at the same level as the person (sitting or standing).
- Speak in a quiet calm tone of voice, limiting eye contact and avoiding changes in voice tone, facial expression, and gestures (especially avoid pointing or waving a finger at the person).
- Ask the person's name (if necessary) and use the name when addressing the person.
- Validate the person by acknowledging their issue: "I can see that you are angry about the changes in your treatment."
- Show empathy without being judgmental: "I'm sorry you are upset."
- Ignore questions that are challenging and avoid arguing.
- Practice active listening by paraphrasing and clarifying.
- Assist the person to explore options and the results of those options: "What is it that you would like to do?"

Geriatric Pathophysiology

GERIATRIC SYNDROMES

Geriatric syndromes represent a category of illnesses that is comprised of the most common non-disease conditions that are seen amongst the geriatric community. It is the responsibility of the nurse to be competent in these critical areas:

- **Falls**: As individuals age, their senses dull, leaving them vulnerable to falls due to a combination of sensory decline and chronic disease. Patients and caregivers should be provided with recommendations for fall prevention, and health care providers should create safe inpatient environments with proper fall prevention protocols.

- **Frailty**: A syndrome characterized by decreased stamina, strength, weight, and speed. This combination of issues results from the natural decline of aging and presents specific risks (falls, confusion, and depression) that must be assessed amongst the geriatric population.
- **Incontinence**: Urinary incontinence is an especially common ailment amongst the elderly population due to neurological conditions, physical limitations, and cognitive decline. This particular ailment is not only physically limiting and introduces risks for skin breakdown and infection, but it is socially limiting and can lead to psychological issues as well.
- **Delirium**: Confusion is the most common manifestation of any physical ailment amongst the elderly, along with the prevalence of dementia amongst the elderly. Delirium should never be cast aside in an elderly individual. Though common, it may be an indication of other more serious issues.
- **Functional Decline**: Functional decline is the diminished ability of an individual to carry out the activities of daily living to sustain independence and perform self-care. With this, comes the consideration for additional support, be it live-in care, nursing homes, or assisted living communities.

Additional Health Issues for the Elderly

The following are additional health issues for the elderly:

- **Antibodies and Immunity**: An elderly patient can react to an infection with antibodies that have been created by the body before, but if the infection is new, it is more difficult for the body to respond appropriately. Cells in the immune system cannot proliferate as easily in an older patient as in a younger one. The number of T-cells is stable, but they do not work as well and can have less cytotoxicity. Additionally, there is not as much thymus-gained immunity because the thymus gland is smaller. This also means it is harder for an older patient to make antibodies.
- **Allergies**: Identify the type of allergic response the patient has and to what allergens, especially when getting the patient history. Determine if the response is actually an allergy to a medication or an adverse effect of it.
- **Driving**: An elderly patient senses change with age. A decreased ability to hear does not mean a patient cannot drive, but sight is very important, including binocular sight, ability to see color, and ability to see in the dark.
- **REM**: Rapid eye movement starts approximately 120 minutes after going to sleep, and happens again in 3–4 evenly spread out increments that last 10–15 minutes. It is linked to skeletal muscle atonia, rapid eye movements, and dreaming. REM sleep occurs less frequently as one gets older. With aging, the patient is more likely to wake up, which affects their sleep quality.

Urinary Incontinence

Urinary incontinence (UI) is the involuntary loss of urine. Incidence increases with age and is more common in women. There are several **types of urinary incontinence**:

- **Transient**: Adverse medication reaction, urinary tract infection, severe constipation, immobility, mental disorders.
- **Urge or Reflex**: Detrusor muscle spasms cause an urgent desire to urinate because of neurological impairment in Parkinson's, stroke, Alzheimer's, and sitting. Can be triggered by drinking, or hearing or seeing running water.

- **Stress (SUI)**: Increased intra-abdominal pressure from sneezing, coughing, laughing, pregnancy, childbirth damage to the detrusor muscle and pelvic floor fascia, and menopausal hormone changes. Twice as common in women as men.
- **Enuresis**: Bedwetting while asleep.

Decreased bladder strength, diminished ability to concentrate urine, and decreased urethral closing pressure following menopause are common causes of incontinence in the elderly. Incontinence is also influenced by depression, less mobility, decreased vision, and less awareness of feeling a full bladder. Voiding routines are helpful in managing incontinence among the elderly. The typical voiding routine for a fully-grown adult patient is as follows: The initial urge to go to the bathroom happens at the point of the bladder having 200-300 mL in it. Grown patients generally void 4-6 times daily, and most will not need to go during the night except when there is a condition that makes it so or if the patient is using diuretic medication. The sensation of the bladder beginning to fill up begins at 90-150 mL, and the need to go starts at 200-300 mL. Usually, an hour or two will elapse between the first feeling of needing to go and the bladder being at full capacity. Full, easy capacity is around 300-600 mL. There should not be any leaking if going to the bathroom has to be postponed.

AGE-RELATED CHANGES IN RESPIRATORY SYSTEM

As a patient ages, the respiratory system changes in the following ways:

- **Rib cage becomes more rigid.** There will be more width measured across the anteroposterior chest. When a patient gets old, the number of alveoli decreases. They get inflexible and can no longer draw back. This means that the patient cannot breathe out as well, leading to more residual volume. There is less basilar inflation and the patient cannot get foreign bodies out as well. This condition also happens to someone who has kyphosis.
- **Decreased ability for the chest wall to work** so that it is harder to take a deep inhalation.
- **Trachea and bronchi increase in measurement** so that there is more unused area and lessened air volume that gets to the alveoli. Small airway shutting means there is less vital capacity and more residual volume.
- **Lung parenchyma is not as elastic** so that the alveoli do not function as effectively.
- **Breaths are not as deep and coughs are not as forceful** because the muscles are not as strong.

CHRONIC DIARRHEA

Chronic diarrhea is more than three bowel movements per day, with watery stools lasting more than two weeks. It is more common and potentially more serious for the elderly population. The most common cause is infectious, but **chronic diarrhea** in the elderly population can also be caused by inflammatory bowel disease, diverticulitis, colon cancer, medication side effects, and irritable bowel syndrome. Take a careful history, including a list of travel destinations. Look for these signs and **symptoms of dehydration** in the physical exam:

- Flushed, dry skin
- Dark, scanty urine
- Fast pulse and respiration
- Fever
- Vomiting or nausea
- Head rushes
- Thirst
- Dry mouth

- Anorexia
- Chills
- Tingling
- Cramps
- Exhaustion
- Confusion
- Seizures
- Unconsciousness

Send stools to the lab for culture, ova and parasites, occult blood, fecal leukocytes, and *C. difficile* toxin, especially if the patient was recently hospitalized. Collect blood for a CBC and electrolytes. Order an abdominal x-ray, and follow up with a barium enema or colonoscopy, if indicated. Treat the underlying cause. Significantly dehydrated patients require hospital admission for IV therapy.

Muscle Wasting or Atrophy

Sarcopenia describes the process of progressive muscle wasting that is seen in the elderly population. Muscle protein production decreases with age, resulting in a loss of muscle mass, and eventually a loss of physical functional ability. Decreased activity and a lack of exercise contribute to the process of muscle wasting. As sarcopenia progresses, it leads to decreased mobility and puts patients at higher risk for developing other health problems. The process of muscle wasting can be slowed, halted, or reversed with treatment. The most effective treatment is exercise, specifically resistance training. Adequate nutrition, including sufficient amounts of Vitamin B_{12}, protein, and calcium is an important part of the treatment regimen. Use of growth hormone, estrogen or testosterone is controversial. Sarcopenia differs from **cachexia**, which is wasting from a chronic disease, most often cancer.

Fractures

Fractures are a common cause of disability in the elderly population. The elderly population is at higher risk for sustaining **fractures** due to decreased bone mass and strength, and increased risk for falls due to poor vision and balance. The most common locations for fractures in the elderly are the distal radius, proximal humerus, proximal femur and tibia, vertebrae, hip, and pubic ramus. Most fractures are the result of minor trauma. Fractures are slightly more common in women. Make the diagnosis based on the history, physical exam, and x-ray results. Immobilize the fracture above and below the break. Administer analgesics. Refer the patient to a physiotherapist, an orthopedic surgeon, and a PSW. The goal of treatment is as rapid a return to normal activity as is possible. The elderly population is more vulnerable to complications, such as permanent functional impairment, bedsores, and pulmonary embolism. The aide, nurse, or caregiver must turn the patient every two hours to minimize complications.

Age-Related Cataracts

The lens is the clear part of the eye behind the pupil that focuses light on the retina. **Cataracts** are categorized by gradual clouding or opacification of the lens. One or both eyes can be affected, and cataracts can be congenital. Incidence increases with age and affects 70% of people over the age of 75. Risk factors include trauma, radiation, diabetes, family history, smoking, alcoholism, sun exposure, steroid use, and previous eye surgery. Signs and symptoms for cataracts include gradual lens clouding; blurry vision; decreased night vision; brown tint or color fading; halo or glare around lights; diplopia (double vision); trouble distinguishing blue and purple. An ophthalmologist makes the diagnosis by slit lamp exam and retinal exam. Cataracts are followed until they cause significant visual loss and then are treated by surgical removal of the clouded lens and replacement with a permanent intraocular or removable external lens.

Hearing Loss

Approximately 25% of adults over the age of 65 have varying degrees of hearing loss. Risk factors for hearing loss include:

- A positive family history
- Chronic exposure to loud noises, especially if hearing protection was not worn
- Use of ototoxic drugs, like Gentamicin, NSAIDs, loop diuretics, or cancer chemotherapy

Hearing loss can be either peripheral or central. **Peripheral hearing loss** results when the ear canal is obstructed by impacted wax, a foreign object, or damage to the middle or inner ear. **Central hearing loss** is the result of damage to the portions of the brain that are needed for hearing: Vestibulocochlear nerve, brain stem, contralateral inferior colliculus, superior olivary nucleus, inferior colliculi, ipsilateral medial geniculate nucleus of the thalamus, and primary auditory cortex below the superior temporal gyrus in the temporal lobe.

Sinusitis

Elderly individuals are at higher risk for the development of **sinusitis**. Causes include the drying out of the nasal passages, weakened nasal cartilage leading to obstruction, and a weakened immune system. The elderly population is also at increased risk for more severe infections and complications. Sinusitis can be acute or chronic. It is considered acute if symptoms have been present for less than four weeks. Patients usually present with fever, cough, facial pain, headache, mouth breathing, and nasal discharge. The diagnosis is generally made clinically; however, occasionally a CT scan and nasal swab for culture and sensitivity can be helpful. Treatment includes antibiotics and decongestants. Chronic sinusitis requires a referral to an ENT specialist (otorhinolaryngologist).

Hypogonadism

Male **hypogonadism** means that the testes do not produce sufficient quantities of testosterone. The patient will be impotent, infertile, and have little or no sex drive. Male hypogonadism can be present at birth from Klinefelter or Kallmann syndromes, and may present also with a micropenis and/or undescended testicles. Hypogonadism can occur later in life from pituitary or testicular tumors, especially if the man must be castrated (orchiectomy) to slow advancing prostate cancer. Hypogonadism results from aging in 30% of men over the age of 50 as **andropause**. Patients present with beard and body hair loss, decreased muscle mass, osteoporosis, gynecomastia (female pattern breast growth), and complain of erectile dysfunction (ED), emotional lability, fatigue, inability to concentrate, and decreased libido. Patients may also have hot flashes. The diagnosis is made based on the clinical picture and the serum testosterone level. Treatment is testosterone replacement therapy, but it can cause polycythemia. A good serum testosterone target level for seniors is 250-1,000 ng/dL.

Menopause

Menopause is cessation of menstrual cycles and childbearing. It is diagnosed after a woman has no periods for 12 *consecutive* months. Perimenopausal women skip periods for months but are not infertile. Menopause is usually a natural process of normal ageing. However, many women experience instant menopause through complete hysterectomy (TAHBSO), cancer chemotherapy, radiation exposure, early ovarian failure, or another pathological condition. The average age of menopause is 51; normal age range is 45-55. Late menopause is 60 and is a risk for uterine cancer. Symptoms of impending menopause include irregular periods, hot flashes, emotional lability, and difficulty sleeping because of night sweats. Diagnosis is made clinically, and confirmed with blood tests for LH, FSH, estrogen, and thyroid panel. The onset of menopause produces an elevated follicle-stimulating hormone level and a decreased estradiol level. Treatment is combined estrogen and progesterone replacement therapy, antidepressants, gabapentin, and clonidine. Do not use estrogen alone if the woman still has her uterus, because it predisposes her to cancer.

Common Comorbidities Seen Amongst the Elderly Population

Geriatric comorbidities are combinations of chronic or acute illnesses that significantly increase the mortality rate amongst this population and are also associated with faster rates of disability exacerbation and functional decline. Understanding these comorbidities not only help the nurse manage these specific comorbidities, but also aid in the guidance of health promotion and disease prevention efforts to decrease the rates of comorbidity amongst their elderly patients. A 2010 study clustered comorbidities most commonly found in the elderly population into 3 groups (Ross, 2010). The three most common comorbidity patterns amongst the geriatric population include:

- **Cardiovascular/Metabolic Disorders**: Heart disease, MI, coronary artery disease and congestive heart failure often coincide with metabolic issues such as hypertension, diabetes, obesity, and gout.
- **Anxiety/Depression/Somatoform Disorders and Pain**: Pain (systemic, localized, or joint related) often coincide with psychological conditions such as anxiety, depression, and cognitive decline. Gastrointestinal issues also seem to coincide with these psychological conditions.
- **Neuropsychiatric Disorders**: Psychiatric conditions such as Parkinson's and dementia, are often tied to neurological issues such as incontinence, vascular issues, and/or nerve pain.

Common Psychological Responses to Chronic Illness

Chronic illness not only effects the physical health of individuals, but often has many **psychological manifestations** as well. This psychological stress is tied to the most basic needs that are engrained in individuals as children, and therefore can cause the regression of the patient to adapt more childlike responses to chronic illness over time. Often these psychological responses to chronic illnesses are based on general concepts of fear, self-esteem, and loss of control.

- **Fear**: Chronic illness, when debilitating with possibly severe consequences, forces patients to face common fears of death, loss, and pain. Remaining in a constant state of fear (stress) can lead to depression, anxiety, and anger.
- **Self Esteem**: While in the early stages of chronic illness many patients find strength and determination to conquer the disease. But, after time, the inability to do so wears on the individual's sense of strength and capability. With a loss of self-esteem, can come feelings of despair and hopelessness, which often result in an increasing rate of decline. Patients with strong support systems and positive outlooks often fare better with chronic disease.
- **Loss of Control**: When chronic disease dictates an individual's life and abilities, the patient loses a sense of control over their own life. Losing one's independence can be extremely difficult mentally and emotionally, especially when the patient was previously active and healthy. By providing the patient with treatment options and educating the patient on self-care the nurse can attempt to return some elements of control to the patient, which can motivate them to own their fight against disease and find a new normal in their life that is manageable and fulfilling.

Alternative, Complementary, and Non-Pharmacologic Interventions

Complementary Therapy

Complementary therapies are often used, either alone or in conjunction with conventional medical treatment. These methods should be included if this is what the patient/family chooses, empowering the family to take control of their plan of care. Complementary therapies vary widely and most can easily be incorporated. The **National Center for Complementary and Alternative Medicine** recognizes the following:

- **Whole medical systems**: Chinese medicine (acupressure, acupuncture), naturopathic and homeopathic medicines, and Ayurveda
- **Mind-body medicine**: Prayer, artistic creation, music and dance therapy, biofeedback, focused relaxation, and visualization
- **Biological medicine**: Aromatherapy, herbs, plants, trees, vitamins and minerals, and dietary supplements
- **Manipulation**: Massage and spinal manipulation
- **Energy medicines**: Magnets, electric current, pulsed fields, Reiki, qi gong, and laying-on of the hands

Precautions

The use of alternative and complementary therapies should be thoroughly discussed by patients and their physician. Patients should be encouraged to use therapies that are shown to have a beneficial, complementary effect on conventional medical treatment. These therapies include the use of massage, superficial stimulation, relaxation, distraction, hypnosis, and guided imagery.

- Encourage patients to practice the techniques until they are proficient in their use to give them a chance to prove their value.
- Teach the patient how the therapies work to encourage the patient to believe in them to contribute to the placebo effect.
- Caution the patient against abandoning current medical treatment.
- Inform the patient of the high cost of alternate therapies that can divert needed funds and result in little or no benefit.
- Provide the patient with resources in the form of books, pamphlets, and informative websites that prove the results of scientific research so that they can evaluate alternative therapies for themselves.

Whole Medical Systems

Whole medical systems are different philosophies and methods of explaining and treating health and illness. Some systems include:

- **Homeopathic medicine**: This European system uses small amounts of diluted herbs and supplements to help the body to recover from disease by stimulating an immune response.
- **Naturopathic medicine**: This is a European system that uses various natural means (herbs, massage, acupuncture) to support the natural healing forces of the body.
- **Chinese medicine**: Centers on restoring the proper flow of life forces within the body to cure disease by using herbs, acupressure and acupuncture, and meditation.
- **Ayurveda**: This is an Indian system that tries to bring the spirit into harmony with the mind and body to treat disease via yoga, herbs, and massage.

Essential Oils and Cupping

Essential oils (concentrated oils from plants) are either inhaled (aromatherapy) or diluted and applied to the skin. Essential oils are believed to reduce stress, aid sleep, improve dermatitis, and aid digestion. Commonly used essential oils include eucalyptus, lavender, lemon, peppermint, rosemary, rose, and tea tree. Oils may cause skin irritation when applied to the skin.

Cupping is an ancient practice still used in Southeast Asia and the Middle East to reduce pain, promote healing, and improve circulation. With dry cupping, cups are heated by placing something flammable (such as paper or herbs) inside the cup and setting it on fire to heat the cup, which is then immediately placed on the back along the meridians (generally on both sides of the spine) to form a vacuum that draws blood to the skin and causes circular bruises believed to heal that part of the body. Wet cupping includes leaving the heated cup in place for three minutes, removing it, making small cuts in the skin, and then applying suction cups again to withdraw blood. Cupping should be avoided in children under 4 and limited to short periods in older children.

Acupuncture

Alternative systems of medical practice include acupuncture, homeopathy, and naturopathy. **Acupuncture**, an ancient Oriental practice, uses stainless steel or copper needles inserted into superficial skin layers at points where energy or life force called *qi* is believed to occur. The needles are supposed to restore balance and the flow of *qi*. The NIH has recognized the effectiveness of acupuncture for certain side effects of other cancer treatments, such as nausea, vomiting, and pain. However, there is no documented scientific evidence to support the principles expounded. Acupuncturists are certified through either formal coursework or apprenticeships, and there is also board certification in this area for physicians. The needles used are classified as class II, which means they have manufacturing and labeling requirements.

Herbal Remedies and Regulations

In the United States, most **herbal preparations** are classified as dietary supplements. That means that they are not subject to the same rigorous manufacturing, safety, efficacy, and control practices as pharmaceutical drugs. Herbal supplements are only governed by the Dietary Supplement and Health Education Act (DSHEA). As long as no specific disease treatment or curative claims are made, the supplement can be marketed without limitation and safety concerns must be pursued by the FDA after the fact. Nevertheless, some herbal remedies have been undergoing clinical trials in the U.S. to substantiate their health-enhancing or traditional/historical or international use claims. However, the focal point of these studies is still only on the effectiveness of the specific supplement. In Europe, there has been some movement toward greater regulation and licensing of herbal products, but not to the extent of formal drug regulations.

Toxicities Associated with Herbal Remedies

Use of herbal preparations has been associated with a variety of **toxicities**, primarily in categories such as cardiovascular problems, hypersensitivity reactions, disorientation, gastrointestinal problems, and liver malfunction. Because quality control measures are relatively lax for these remedies, contamination from infectious agents and toxic metals can potentially cause other side effects. Many of these herbal medicines **interact with conventional drugs**, thus altering their pharmacodynamics. For example, St. John's wort, which is primarily used for depressive disorders or as a sedative, interacts with a wide range of traditional pharmacologic agents and suppresses their levels in the bloodstream. Kava kava, made from dried roots of a type of pepper bush, is used as a sedative, but it also has been associated with hepatic failure and via interactions with several other drugs can actually induce a comatose state. Ginseng is an Asian remedy touted for its curative properties in a number of diseases. However, it can react with steroidal drugs and induce shaking and manic episodes. These are just a few examples of potential dangers.

NON-PHARMACEUTICAL PAIN RELIEF

Non-pharmaceutical methods to relieve pain that can be used exclusively or combined with medications include massage, heat, cold, electrical stimulation, distraction, relaxation, imagery, visualization, and music. Other **alternatives or adjuncts to pain medication** include hypnosis, magnets, acupuncture, acupressure, and therapeutic touch. Herbs, aromatherapy, reflexology, homeopathic medicine, and prayer may also be accepted by the patient. Any method that the patient feels may help that isn't harmful should be used to help get relief.

MIND-BODY MEDICINE FOR PAIN AND DISEASE

Mind-body medicine (prayer, artistic creation, music and dance, biofeedback, relaxation, and visualization) can help distract people from pain or other symptoms if they are able to concentrate on the method. This can result in the transfer of less painful stimuli to the brain by stimulating the **descending control system**. These methods work if the patient can use them to create alternate sensations in the brain, but will not work if the patient is unable to concentrate due to intense pain.

Relaxation that occurs as a result of using these methods helps to reduce muscular tension that can make pain worse and reduces fatigue caused by chronic pain. Relaxation has been proven to be the most helpful after surgery. Postoperative patients report a greater feeling of control over their pain and tend to request fewer opioids to control pain. Biofeedback can help patients to recognize the feelings of both tension and relaxation and provide a way to indicate their success in managing muscle tension.

USE OF VISUALIZATION

There are a number of methods used for **visualization** to reduce anxiety and promote healing. Some include audiotapes with guided imagery, such as self-hypnosis tapes, but the patient can be taught basic **techniques** that include:

- Sit or lie comfortably in a **quiet place** away from distractions.
- Concentrate on **breathing** while taking long slow breaths.
- **Close the eyes** to shut out distractions and create an image in the mind of the place or situation desired.
- Concentrate on that **image**, engaging as many senses as possible and imaging details.
- If the mind wanders, breathe deeply and **bring consciousness back** to the image or concentrate on breathing for a few moments and then return to the imagery.
- End with positive imagery.

Sometimes, patients are resistive at first or have a hard time maintaining focus, so **guiding** them through visualization for the first few times can be helpful.

STIMULATION OF THE SKIN TO REDUCE PAIN

Skin, muscles, fascia, tendons, and the cornea contain **nociceptors** that are nerve endings that respond to painful stimuli. Massage, transcutaneous electrical nerve stimulation (TENS), heat and cold provide stimulation to other nerves that transfer only sensation, not pain. These signals block some of the transfer of the nociceptor impulses:

- **Massage** not only sends alternate sensation to the brain, but also results in relaxation that decreases the muscular tension that contributes to pain.
- **TENS** works well on incisional and neuromuscular pain by providing a gentle electrical stimulation that overrides the painful impulses from the area and may stimulate endorphins.
- **Heat therapy** increases blood flow and oxygen to promote healing and stimulates neural receptors, decreasing pain. Heat also helps loosen tense muscles that may be contributing to pain.
- **Cold therapy** decreases circulation and reduces production of chemicals related to inflammation, thereby reducing pain.

Temperature-Controlled Therapies
Methods of Heating and Cooling

There are a number of different ways to **heat** (thermotherapy) or **cool** (cryotherapy) for **healing**:

- **Conduction**: Conveyance of heat, cold, or electricity through direct contact with the skin, such as with hot baths, ice packs, and electrical stimulation.
- **Convection**: Indirect transmission of heat in a liquid or gas by circulation of heated particles, such as with whirlpools and paraffin soaks.
- **Conversion**: Heating that results from converting a form of energy into heat, such as with diathermy and ultrasound.
- **Evaporation**: Cooling caused by liquids that evaporate into gases on the skin with a resultant cooling effect, such as with perspiration or vapo-coolant sprays.
- **Radiation**: Heating that results from transfer of heat through light waves or rays, such as with infrared or ultraviolet light.

Shortwave Diathermy

Shortwave diathermy uses radio waves (27.12 megahertz) to **increase the temperature in subcutaneous tissue** and is used along with passive and active range of motion exercises to **improve range** in painful conditions such as inflammation of the muscles, tendons, and bursae. The radio waves (eddy currents) are transmitted through a capacitor or inductor in a continuous or pulse waveform. Temperatures increase about 15 °C in fatty tissue and 4-6 °C in muscular tissue. Shortwave diathermy should not be used over any organs containing fluid, including the eyes, heart, head, or over pacemakers as the diathermy may disrupt the settings. Because this treatment may increase cardiac demand, it should be avoided in those with preexisting cardiac conditions and should not be used over malignancies. Additionally, it is contraindicated in areas of inflammation because heating the tissue increases inflammation. It cannot be used over prostheses as the metal may heat and damage tissue. Shortwave diathermy should avoid the epiphyses in children, as it may stimulate abnormal growth.

Microwave Diathermy

Microwave diathermy is used similarly to shortwave diathermy but has a lower rate of heat increase and penetrance so it is used for muscles and joints near the surface rather than deep muscles, such as the hip. Heat is created by **electromagnetic radiation** (9.15-14.50 MHz) and raises temperature in fatty tissues by about 10-12 °C and in muscular tissue by 3-4 °C. **Treatment** is usually given for 15-30 minutes per session and is followed by range of motion exercises (passive and active) to increase flexibility. Contraindications are similar to those of shortwave diathermy in that this treatment should not be used where increase in temperature may be detrimental, such as over organs containing fluid, areas of inflammation, and epiphyses of children. Additionally, it should not be used over prostheses or pacemakers and should be avoided in those with cardiac disease.

SUPERFICIAL HEAT

Superficial heat with externally applied heat sources penetrates only the superficial layers of the skin (1-2 cm after about 30 minutes), but it is believed to relax deeper muscles by reflex, decrease pain, and increase metabolisms (2-3 times for every 10 °C increase in skin temperature). Therapeutic temperature range is 40-45 °C. **Superficial heat modalities** include:

- **Moist heat packs** placed on the skin and secured by several layers of towels to provide insulation, applied for 15-30 minutes.
- **Paraffin baths** (52-54 °C) with the hand, foot, or elbow dipped 7 times, cooling between dippings, and then wrapping with plastic and towels for 20 minutes.
- **Fluidotherapy** uses hot-air warmed (38.8-47.8 °C) cellulose particles into which a hand or foot is submerged for 20-30 minutes.

Passive and active range of motion exercises are done after superficial heat treatment. Contraindications include cardiac disease, peripheral vascular disease, malignant tumor, bleeding, and acute inflammation.

Deep heat differs from superficial heat in that the heat is generated internally using ultrasound, short wave, and microwave diathermy rather than applied to the surface of the skin. Deep heating has penetrance to 3-5 cm.

CRYOTHERAPY

Cryotherapy uses therapeutic cold treatment to cool the surface of the skin and underlying subcutaneous tissues in order to decrease blood flow, pain, and metabolism. Initially response to cold therapy causes **vasoconstriction** to occur within the first 15 minutes but if the tissues are cooled to -10 °C, then the body responds with **vasodilation**. Cryotherapy affects sensory response so the person will at first feel cold, which progresses to burning, aching, and finally to numbness and tingling. Treatment is usually given for 15-30 minutes. **Treatment modalities** include:

- **Ice packs** such as refrigerated gel packs (-5 °C) or plastic bags filled with water and ice chips are applied directly to the skin for 10-15 minutes for superficial cooling and 15-20 minutes for greater penetrance.
- A **towel dipped in ice and water slurry** is wrapped around limb to provide cold therapy, but this is best used only for emergency situations when ice packs are unavailable, as the towel must be changed frequently as the skin warms the towel rapidly.
- **Ice massage** is applied directly to the affected area for 5-10 minutes, usually rubbing the ice in circular motions on the skin surface. An ice massager is easily made by filled a paper cup with water and freezing it with a tongue depressor or Popsicle stick (to use as a handle) inserted into the center as the water starts to freeze. Then, the paper can be torn away from the bottom and sides when the ice is solid. Ice massage is often followed by friction massage.
- **Ice baths** (13-18 °C) are used for limbs, such as the lower leg, foot, or hand. The body part is immersed for 20 minutes.

Cryotherapy is usually followed by **active and passive exercises**. Contraindications include impaired circulation or sensation, cardiac disease, Raynaud's disease, and nerve trauma.

Whirlpool Baths

Whirlpool baths are used to increase **circulation** and promote **healing**. They are tubs with a turbine that mixes air with water, which is pressurized and flows into the tub water to create turbulence. Tubs are usually large enough to accommodate the full body although smaller limb-sized whirlpool tubs are available. Water temperature is 95-104 °F (adjusted for the individual) and should be deep enough to completely submerge the affected part. The body part should be cleaned with soap and water before immersion or a shower taken. If the full body is treated, then the patient should wear a swimming suit. During the whirlpool treatment, the muscles relax from the heat and **range of motion exercises** can be done while in the water. Typically, treatments last about 20 minutes, but the patient should be monitored, especially for the first 5 minutes, as some people become lightheaded and can lose consciousness.

Contrast Baths

Contrast baths (alternating hot and cold) are used in the sub-acute phase of healing (after edema begins to subside) for **strains and sprains**. It is believed that contrast baths increase the circulation and help to further decrease edema by a pumping action as the **vasoconstriction and vasodilation** alternate. Two containers are filled with water, one with hot and the other with cold. The hot water should be maintained at about 100-110 °F and the cold at 55-65 °F. The cycle begins and ends with immersion in cold water. Cold water immersions usually last about 1 minute and hot water immersions 4 minutes. Typically, the affected limb is immersed in the cold water for 1 minute, removed, and immediately immersed in hot water for 4 minutes. This cycle is repeated about 3-4 times.

Therapeutic Ultrasound

Ultrasound treats soft-tissue injuries (such as myositis, bursitis, and tendinitis) with sound waves (frequency 0.8-3 megahertz). Ultrasound utilizes a **piezoelectric crystal** that vibrates, producing sound waveforms, which are transmitted from the transducer through a gel substance into the tissue. The sound waves bounce off of the bone in an irregular pattern that causes an increase in temperature in the connective tissue, such as collagen fibers. Temperatures of the tissue may increase up to 43.5 °C, increasing metabolism in the area, neural conduction, as well as blood flow. Ultrasound is used to **decrease both contractures and scarring**. During treatment, the transducer passes in a circular motion about the skin surface, staying in contact with the gel medium. If a distal limb is submerged in water, the treatment is given with the head of the transducer 0.5-1 inch from the skin surface. Treatment is followed by range of motion exercises, passive and active. Contraindications are similar to other heat-producing modalities and include peripheral vascular disease, but ultrasound may be used over metal prostheses.

TENS

Transcutaneous electrical nerve stimulation (TENS) uses electrical stimulation to stimulate **peripheral sensory nerve fibers** to reduce acute or recurrent pain. TENS machines may be 2-lead or 4-lead and have adjustments for both frequency (1-20 Hz) and pulse width (50-300 microseconds, 10-50 mA). Stimulation can be intermittent or continuous. TENS units are small and battery-powered with wires and adhesive electrodes attached so that they can be worn while the person goes about usual activities. The positioning of the electrodes and the settings depend upon the site and type of injury, following guidelines provided by the manufacturer. The TENS machine can be used for a number of hours, but if used for days at a time, it will be less effective. TENS treatment is contraindicated with demand pacemakers and should not be used on the head or neck or over irritated skin.

Rehabilitation

SAID Principle of Rehabilitation and Reconditioning

The Specific Adaptation to Imposed Demands (SAID) principle suggests that when a person is injured or stressed, that person attempts to overcome the problem by **adapting** to the demands of the situation. This is based on **Wolff's law** (systems adapt to demands). For example, if one hand is not usable, the person adapts and uses the other hand. Unfortunately, this adaptation can lead to increasing disability, so when the SAID principle is applied to rehabilitation, it means that the person must do exercises that specifically aim to correct the problem. Thus, the functional needs of the person should always be considered when designing a specific exercise program for that individual (such as treadmill running for soccer players). The exercise activities should as closely mirror the functional activities as possible. For example, if the goal is increased strength rather than endurance, then the exercise program should rely more heavily on strengthening exercises.

Massage for Rehabilitation and Reconditioning

Massage therapy is commonly used in sports and may be employed before activities, at breaks during activities, and after the activity is completed. Many types of massage are used in sports, and some massage therapists specialize in sports massage, but all nurses who work with athletes of any age should know the basic techniques of **sports massage** as it is used to both treat and prevent injuries. Sports massage is based primarily on Swedish massage although the massage may be deeper and targeted toward a particular injury, and other types of massage may be incorporated into a sports massage program. Massage of an injured area is delayed for the first **48-72 hours** to prevent further injury to tissues. Different techniques include:

- **Compression**: Deep rhythmical compressions of the muscles are done to increase circulation and temperature and make muscles more pliable. It may be used prior to deeper massage techniques.
- **Effleurage**: This is usually the beginning massage and begins softly and increases in intensity with the hands gliding over the tissue, so it is done with some type of oil or emollient. Massage is done in rhythmical broad strokes with the palms of the hands. This massage helps to relax the athlete and identify areas of tightness or pain that may require additional attention.
- **Friction**: These are massages either in line with muscle fibers or across the muscle fibers to create stretching and to reduce adhesions and scarring during healing. The tissue is pressed firmly against the underlying tissue and then pressure moves the underlying tissue until resistance is felt. Friction massage may be done deeply, and this can be uncomfortable. Usually, the thumb or fingers are used for this type of massage
- **Petrissage**: This is kneading massage and is usually used on large muscle areas, such as the calf or thigh. It increases circulation, so it is useful to relax and to improve circulation and drainage as well as to stretch muscles. The full hand is used for this massage with the heel and thumb stabilizing the tissue while the fingers squeeze the tissue.
- **Tapotement**: This type of massage uses quick rhythmic tapping, usually with the edge of the palm and little finger or the heel of the hand with the fingers elevated. It is done to increase circulation or relieve cramped muscles.
- **Vibration**: Vibratory massage is used for deep muscle relaxation and reduction of pain. Usually, the entire hand is placed against the skin, compressing the muscle and then vibrating the hand to cause movement.
- **Trigger point**: Pressure is applied with a finger or thumb to areas of point tenderness to reduce spasticity and pain.

PROGRESSION IN STRENGTHENING EXERCISES

Strengthening exercise progression includes the following exercises:

- **Isometric exercises** are done with the muscle and limb in static position with no movement of the joint or lengthening of the muscle. The muscle is contracted against resistance.
- **Isotonic exercises** include movement of the joint during exercise (such as running, weight lifting) and both shortening and lengthening of the muscles through eccentric or concentric contractions. Isotonic refers to tension, so the tension is constant during shortening and lengthening of the muscle.
- **Isokinetic exercises** utilize machines (such as stationary bicycles that can be set with various parameters) to control the rate and extent of contraction as well as the range of motion. Both speed and resistance can be set so the athlete is limited by the settings of the machine.
- **Plyometrics** is a particular type of exercise program that uses activities to allow a muscle to achieve maximal force as quickly as possible, and the sequence is a fast, eccentric movement (to stretch) followed quickly by a strong concentric movement (to contract).

Care Coordination and Collaboration

SKILLS NEEDED FOR COLLABORATION

Nurses must learn the set of skills needed for **collaboration** in order to move nursing forward. Nurses must take an active role in gathering data for evidence-based practice to support nursing's role in health care, and they must share this information with other nurses and health professionals in order to plan staffing levels and to provide optimal care to patients. Increased and adequate staffing has consistently been shown to reduce adverse outcomes, but there is a well-documented shortage of nurses in the United States, and more than half of current RNs work outside the hospital. Increased patient loads not only increase adverse outcomes but also increase job dissatisfaction and burnout. In order to manage the challenges facing nursing, nurses must develop the following skills needed for collaboration:

- Be willing to compromise
- Communicate clearly
- Identify specific challenges and problems
- Focus on the task
- Work with teams

COMMUNICATION SKILLS

Collaboration requires a number of communication skills that differ from those involved in communication between nurse and patient. These skills include:

- **Using an assertive approach:** It's important for the nurse to honestly express opinions and to state them clearly and with confidence, but the nurse must do so in a calm, non-threatening manner.
- **Making casual conversation:** It's easier to communicate with people with whom one has a personal connection. Asking open-ended questions, asking about other's work, or commenting on someone's contributions helps to establish a relationship. The time before meetings, during breaks, and after meetings presents an opportunity for this type of conversation.

- **Being competent in public speaking:** Collaboration requires that a nurse be comfortable speaking and presenting ideas to groups of people. Speaking and presenting ideas competently also helps the nurse to gain credibility. Public speaking is a skill that must be practiced.
- **Communicating in writing:** The written word remains a critical component of communication, and the nurse should be able to communicate clearly and grammatically.

COMMUNICATION AND HAND OFFS

The nurse is usually the primary staff member responsible for **external and internal hand off transitions of care**, and should ensure that communication is thorough and covers all essential information. The best method is to use a standardized format:

- **DRAW**: Diagnosis, recent changes, anticipated changes, and what to watch for.
- **I PASS the BATON**: Introduction, patient, assessment, situation, safety concerns, background, actions, timing, ownership, and next.
- **ANTICipate**: Administrative data, new clinical information, tasks, illness severity, contingency plans.
- **5 Rs**: Record, review, round together, relay to team, and receive feedback.

A reporting **form** or checklist may be utilized to ensure that no aspect is overlooked.

For external transitions, the nurse must ensure that the type of transport team and monitoring is appropriate for patient needs, and provide insight when determining the most appropriate mode of transportation: ground transfer for short distance, helicopter for medium to long distance, and fixed-wing aircraft for long distances.

SBAR TECHNIQUE

The **SBAR technique** is used to hand-off a patient from one caregiver to another to provide a systematic method so that important information is conveyed:

- **(S) Situation**: Overview of current situation and important issues
- **(B) Background**: Important history and issues leading to current situation
- **(A) Assessment**: Summary of important facts and condition
- **(R) Recommendation**: Actions needed

SHIFT REPORTING

Shift reporting should include bedside handoff when possible with oncoming staff members. The nurse handing off the patient should follow a specific format for handoff (such as I PASS the BATON) so that handoff is done in the same manner every time, as this reduces the chance of omitting important information. The shift report should include introduction of the oncoming staff to the patient, the triage category or acuity level of the patient, diagnosis (potential or confirmed), current status, laboratory and imaging (completed or pending) and results if available, and medications or treatments administered and pending. Any monitoring equipment (pulse oximetry, telemetry) should be examined. Any invasive treatments (Foley catheter, IV) should be discussed and equipment examined. The nurse should report any plans for admission, transfer, or discharge. It is essential that all staff be trained in shift reporting and the importance of consistency.

COLLABORATION BETWEEN NURSE AND PATIENT/FAMILY

One of the most important forms of **collaboration** is that between the nurse and the patient/family, but this type of collaboration is often overlooked. Nurses and others in the healthcare team must always remember that the point of collaboration is to improve patient care, and this means that the patient and patient's family must remain central to all planning. For example, including family in planning for a patient takes time initially, but sitting down and asking the patient and family, "What do you want?" and using the Synergy model to evaluate patient's (and family's) characteristics can provide valuable information that saves time in the long run and facilitates planning and expenditure of resources. Families, and even young children, often want to participate in care and planning and feel validated and more positive toward the medical system when they are included.

COLLABORATION WITH EXTERNAL AGENCIES

The nurse must initiate and facilitate collaboration with **external agencies** because many have direct impacts on patient care and needs:

- **Industry** can include other facilities sharing interests in patient care or pharmaceutical companies. It's important for nursing to have a dialog with drug companies about their products and how they are used in specific populations because many medications are prescribed to women, children, or the aged without validating studies for dose or efficacy.
- **Payers** have a vested interest in containing health care costs, so providing information and representing the interests of the patient is important.
- **Community groups** may provide resources for patients and families, both in terms of information and financial or other assistance.
- **Political agencies** are increasingly important as new laws are considered about nurse-patient ratios and infection control in many states.
- **Public health agencies** are partners in health care with other facilities and must be included, especially in issues related to communicable disease.

INTERDISCIPLINARY TEAMS

There are a number of skills that are needed to lead and facilitate coordination of **intra- and inter-disciplinary teams:**

- Communicating openly is essential. All members must be encouraged to participate as valued members of a cooperative team.
- Avoiding interrupting or interpreting the point another is trying to make allows free flow of ideas.
- Avoiding jumping to conclusions, which can effectively shut off communication.
- Active listening requires paying attention and asking questions for clarification rather than to challenge other's ideas.
- Respecting others opinions and ideas, even when opposed to one's own, is absolutely essential.
- Reacting and responding to facts rather than feelings allows one to avoid angry confrontations and diffuse anger.
- Clarifying information or opinions stated can help avoid misunderstandings.
- Keeping unsolicited advice out of the conversation shows respect for others and allows them to solicit advice without feeling pressured.

LEADERSHIP STYLES

Leadership styles often influence the perception of leadership values and commitment to collaboration. There are a number of different **leadership styles**:

- **Charismatic:** Relies on personal charisma to influence people, and may be very persuasive, but this type leader may engage followers and relate to one group rather than the organization at large, limiting effectiveness.
- **Bureaucratic:** Follows organization rules exactly and expects everyone else to do so. This is most effective in handling cash flow or managing work in dangerous work environments. This type of leadership may engender respect but may not be conducive to change.
- **Autocratic:** Makes decisions independently and strictly enforces rules. Team members often feel left out of process and may not be supportive of the decisions that are made. This type of leadership is most effective in crisis situations, but may have difficulty gaining the commitment of staff.
- **Consultative:** Presents a decision and welcomes input and questions, although decisions rarely change. This type of leadership is most effective when gaining the support of staff is critical to the success of proposed changes.
- **Participatory:** Presents a potential decision and then makes final decision based on input from staff or teams. This type of leadership is time-consuming and may result in compromises that are not entirely satisfactory to management or staff, but this process is motivating to staff who feel their expertise is valued.
- **Democratic:** Presents a problem and asks staff or teams to arrive at a solution, although the leader usually makes the final decision. This type of leadership may delay decision-making, but staff and teams are often more committed to the solutions because of their input.
- **Laissez-faire ("Free Reign"):** Exerts little direct control but allows employees/teams to make decisions with little interference. This may be effective leadership if teams are highly skilled and motivated, but in many cases, this type of leadership is the product of poor management skills and little is accomplished because of this lack of leadership.

TEAM BUILDING

Leading, facilitating, and participating in performance improvement teams requires a thorough understanding of the dynamics of **team building:**

- **Initial interactions:** This is the time when members begin to define their roles and develop relationships, determining if they are comfortable in the group.
- **Power issues:** The members observe the leader and determine who controls the meeting and how control is exercised, beginning to form alliances.
- **Organizing:** Methods to achieve work are clarified and team members begin to work together, gaining respect for each other's contributions and working toward a common goal.
- **Team identification:** Interactions often become less formal as members develop rapport, and members are more willing to help and support each other to achieve goals.
- **Excellence:** This develops through a combination of good leadership, committed team members, clear goals, high standards, external recognition, spirit of collaboration, and a shared commitment to the process.

Team Meetings

Leading and facilitating improvement teams requires utilizing good **techniques for meetings**. Considerations include:

- **Scheduling**: Both the time and the place must be convenient and conducive to working together, so the leader must review the work schedules of those involved, finding the most convenient time. Venues or meeting rooms should allow for sitting in a circle or around a table to facilitate equal exchange of ideas. Any necessary technology, such as computers or overhead projectors, or other equipment, such as whiteboards, should be available.
- **Preparation**: The leader should prepare a detailed agenda that includes a list of items for discussion.
- **Conduction**: Each item of the agenda should be discussed, soliciting input from all group members. Tasks should be assigned to individual members based on their interest and part in the process in preparation for the next meeting. The leader should summarize input and begin a tentative future agenda.
- **Observation**: The leader should observe the interactions, including verbal and nonverbal communication, and respond to them.

Common Vision

Facilitating the creation of a common vision for care within the healthcare system begins with the organization/facility, working collaboratively to create teams and an organization focused on serving the patient/family. A common vision should be the ideal in any organization, but achieving such a goal requires a true collaborative effort:

- Inclusion of all levels of staff across the organization/facility, both those in nursing and non-nursing positions
- Consensus building through discussions, inservice, and team meetings to bring about convergence of diverse viewpoints
- Facilitation that values creativity and provides encouragement during the process
- Vision statement incorporating the common vision that is accessible to all staff
- Recognition that a common vision is an organic concept that may evolve over time and should be reevaluated regularly and changed as needed to reflect the needs of the organization, patients, families, and staff

Facilitating Change

Performance improvement processes cannot occur without organizational change, and **resistance to change** is common for many people, so coordinating collaborative processes requires anticipating resistance and taking steps to achieve cooperation. Resistance often relates to concerns about job loss, increased responsibilities, and general denial or lack of understanding and frustration. Leaders can prepare others involved in the process of change by taking these steps:

- Be honest, informative, and tactful, giving people thorough information about anticipated changes and how the changes will affect them, including positives.
- Be patient in allowing people the time they need to contemplate changes and express anger or disagreement.
- Be empathetic in listening carefully to the concerns of others.
- Encourage participation, allowing staff to propose methods of implementing change, so they feel some sense of ownership.

- Establish a climate in which all staff members are encouraged to identify the need for change on an ongoing basis.
- Present further ideas for change to management.

Conflict Resolution

Conflict is an almost inevitable product of teamwork, and the leader must assume responsibility for **conflict resolution.** While conflicts can be disruptive, they can produce positive outcomes by opening dialogue and forcing team members to listen to different perspectives. The team should make a plan for dealing with conflict. The best time for conflict resolution is when differences emerge but before open conflict and hardening of positions occur. The leader must pay close attention to the people and problems involved, listen carefully, and reassure those involved that their points of view are understood. Steps to conflict resolution include:

- Allow both sides to present their side of conflict without bias, maintaining a focus on opinions rather than individuals.
- Encourage cooperation through negotiation and compromise.
- Maintain the focus, providing guidance to keep the discussions on track and avoid arguments.
- Evaluate the need for re-negotiation, formal resolution process, or third-party involvement.
- Utilize humor and empathy to diffuse escalating tensions.
- Summarize the issues, outlining key arguments.
- Avoid forcing resolution if possible.

Healthcare Team Members

Role of Nursing Care to Support Therapies Provided by Other Disciplines

Nursing care often involves providing **support to therapies** provided by other disciplines. The nurse works as a team member with physicians, occupational and physical therapists, respiratory therapists, social workers, and discharge planners. Floor nurses may work with nurses in other specializations, such as critical care or psychiatric nurses. As a primary coordinator of the care plan, the nurse ensures that the necessary therapies from all disciplines are administered as ordered, and maintains clear communication with all members of the patient's healthcare team. Nurses also support nutritional services by assuring that the patient receives the proper diet for the particular medical or surgical condition, and they communicate with housekeeping to ensure that the patient's environment is appropriate.

Occupational Therapy

The function of occupational therapy is to enable the patient to attain functional outcomes that enhance health, prevent further injury or impairment, and sustain or improve the highest attainable level of independence. The occupational therapist's role is to **facilitate interventions** that aid the patient in improving basic motor and cognitive skills and to **introduce strategies** for meeting challenges at work or at home. In cases of permanent disability or loss of mobility, the occupational therapist works with the patient on adaptive measures to improve function and the ability to perform daily living tasks. Occupational therapists may use physical exercises to improve muscle strength, balance, and dexterity, or cognitive exercises and strategies to improve problem-solving and memory. They help patients with disabilities or cognitive impairments adapt to particular environments, such as a private home or workplace, and teach patients how to use adaptive equipment like wheelchairs, orthotic devices, or computer programs.

Respiratory Therapy

The function of respiratory therapy is to provide care to patients with **respiratory and cardiopulmonary disorders**. The role of the respiratory therapist is to diagnose, evaluate, and treat patients with these disorders, and manage their therapeutic care. The respiratory therapist administers aerosolized medications and provides bronchopulmonary hygiene and postural drainage therapy. The role of the respiratory therapist is also to provide support for mechanically-ventilated patients and to maintain an artificial or natural airway. Many respiratory therapists perform pulmonary function testing as well as hemodynamic monitoring. Some respiratory therapists obtain arterial blood gases and other blood samples, as well as assemble and maintain respiratory equipment. They also teach patients how to self-administer aerosol medications and use life-support respiratory equipment in the home environment.

Case Manager

The case manager is an RN that works for a healthcare insurer as a **manager of the provision of healthcare services** to the people the company insures. One manager or a group of managers are given a caseload of patients with the same range of diagnoses. The case manager is an expert in the range of diagnoses and coordinates services to fulfill the healthcare needs of that particular group of patients. The patient is followed throughout the continuum of care to ensure quality and cost-effectiveness of treatments and care. Complications are prevented and the incidence of repeat hospitalization is decreased. The case manager utilizes evidence-based pathways, clinical pathways, or other plans to track the care and progress of the patient. They are the ones who precertify care, negotiate for payment, and authorize treatment. Patient progress reports from the hospital utilization review or other liaison to the case manager are required at periodic intervals during the hospital stay.

Identifying the Need for Patient Referral

Issues to consider when making patient referrals include:

- **Necessity**: The referral may be needed if the patient's needs are outside of the provider's scope or practice or field of expertise and if the provider cannot provide adequate assessment and treatment for the patient's condition.
- **Insurance requirements**: The provider should determine whether the patient's carrier requires preauthorization or other steps to make sure the patient's referral is covered.
- **Selection of specialist/therapist**: The specialist, in many cases, must be selected from a group of physicians who are participating in an insurance plan if the service is to be covered completely or at all by the insurance company. When possible, the patient should be given choice of referrals.
- **Submission**: The referral should be sent along with appropriate records and releases. The provider may need to make personal contact if specialists are selective, have waiting lists, and may not approve a referral.

Five Rights of Delegation

Prior to delegating tasks, the nurse should assess the needs of the patients and determine the task that needs to be completed, assure that he/she can remain accountable and can supervise the task appropriately, and evaluate effective completion. The **5 rights of delegation** include:

- **Right task:** The nurse should determine an appropriate task to delegate for a specific patient. This would not include tasks that require assessment or planning.
- **Right circumstance:** The nurse has considered the setting, resources, time factors, safety factors, and all other relevant information to determine the appropriateness of delegation. A task that is usually in one's scope (such as feeding a patient) may require assessment that makes it inappropriate to delegate (feeding a new stroke patient).
- **Right person:** The nurse is in the right position to choose the right person (by virtue of education/skills) to perform a task for the right patient.
- **Right direction:** The nurse provides a clear description of the task, the purpose, any limits, and expected outcomes.
- **Right supervision:** The nurse is able to supervise, intervene as needed, and evaluate performance of the task.

Delegation of Tasks in Teams

On major responsibility of leadership and management in performance improvement teams is using **delegation** effectively. The purpose of having a team is so that the work is shared, and leaders can cripple themselves by taking on too much of the workload. Additionally, failure to delegate shows an inherent distrust in team members. Delegation includes:

- Assessing the skills and available time of the team members, determining if a task is suitable for an individual
- Assigning tasks, with clear instructions that include explanation of objectives and expectations, including a timeline
- Ensuring that the tasks are completed properly and on time by monitoring progress but not micromanaging
- Reviewing the final results and recording outcomes

Because the leader is ultimately responsible for the delegated work, mentoring, monitoring, and providing feedback and intervention as necessary during this process is a necessary component of leadership. Even when delegated tasks are not completed successfully, they represent an opportunity for learning.

Telehealth

Telehealth Nursing

Telehealth nursing is a process that provides nursing care for patients over the telephone or other medium of non-physical interaction. Through telehealth services, patients are able to call in and speak with nurses about their symptoms or current condition, and in turn, telehealth nurses can provide health information and guidance to patients without seeing them in person. In addition to phone calls, these visits may also be conducted through videoconferencing, the internet, or other types of media. Some nurses who perform case management services for clients may also utilize telehealth to contact patients and review their current states of health. This type of technology allows these nurses to make assessments with the information provided from the patient, and to then compare these data with former conversations or visits to determine if the patient is moving toward expected outcomes in management of illness.

Necessary Skills

The nurse must master certain skills in order to be able to provide quality care via telehealth:

- The nurse must have excellent **verbal skills** and be able to effectively communicate over the phone to meet patient needs.
- The nurse must have a knowledge of **cultural differences** and be competent in communicating by telephone with patients of different cultures.
- The nurse must be able to **prioritize** the needs of the patient, using the standards of care provided by the *Telehealth Nursing Standards of Practice*, most recently revised in 2017.
- The nurse must be able to **perform** telehealth nursing in a variety of environments, including, but not limited to, clinics, physician's offices, emergency departments, and call centers.
- The nurse must be able to **ask specific questions** that will lead to the optimum treatment plan for the patient and assist in triaging for both nonemergent and emergent states of health.

Telephone Triage

Telephone triage is the process in which the receiving nurse uses protocols and guidelines to assess and prioritize the needs of a patient as they describe their condition over the phone. Telehealth does not allow the nurse to physically see the patient, so the nurse must be skilled at asking the appropriate questions and prioritizing needs based on the patients responses. The nurse must develop a plan of care that may include education, wellness promotion, and preventative education. The telehealth nurse is an extension of the clinic; therefore, he or she must also advocate for the patient and provide additional emotional support. Telehealth nursing increases patient satisfaction by providing the patient with a reliable source of information, direction, and emotional support.

Algorithms

In the telehealth process, patients are guided through triage questions to help the nurse reach a decision for care. **Algorithms** may be used as part of protocol for this triage process. Algorithms are a set of rules designed to solve a certain problem. They are different than a guideline because algorithms direct the nurse toward the best line of treatment. Algorithms also provide a systematic way to evaluate a broad problem or issue. They cover six areas of evaluation, which include the following:

- Assessment and data collection.
- Classification of acuity.
- Degree of advice or intervention.
- Education of caller.
- Validation of the caller.
- Evaluation/Follow-up.

The process follows a chain of logic and relies on the nurse's ability to assess, analyze, and interpret the patient's responses to questions posed by the nurse. The nurse may use algorithms as a direct line of questioning with "yes or no" answers. Each answer directs the nurse to the next type of question, ultimately guiding the nurse to the appropriate way to manage the situation by ruling out other conditions. The use of algorithms in telehealth nursing helps nurses to effectively triage patients over the phone, thereby potentially reducing the frequency of unnecessary emergency department visits and elevated costs.

EFFICIENT USE OF PROTOCOLS OR GUIDELINES

Protocols and guidelines in telehealth provide structure to the assessment process tailored to the patient's symptoms. They help to promote quality care when followed universally by telehealth nurses. Universal guidelines ensure that no matter where a patient lives, he or she is getting information based on the universal nursing standards of care. Some guidelines may be used to educate the patient on upcoming procedures such as ocular exams or hearing tests. Preoperative instructions can also be given through telehealth using standardized guidelines, as are post-hospitalization follow-up instructions. Guidelines are symptom-based and do not require a confirmed medical diagnosis. For example, if a patient calls in with a suspected sprain or break to the leg, the telehealth nurse would refer to the guideline for care that applies to an injury to an extremity (more generally). The nurse must listen carefully to what a patient is saying, but also to what is not being said in order to carefully prioritize the symptoms the patient is describing.

NECESSARY PROFESSIONAL COMPETENCIES AND PROFESSIONAL DEVELOPMENT

As with nurses in any other specialty, telehealth nurses must demonstrate professional nursing competencies and an ongoing knowledge of health care practices. They must show clinical expertise with the populations they serve. **Professional competencies** for the telehealth nurse include the following:

- A knowledge of health and illness across all age groups.
- Assessment skills specific for telephone triage.
- Communication skills, both verbal and written.
- Assertiveness and excellent listening skills.
- Critical thinking skills and effectiveness at educating patients over the phone.
- Customer service skills, including the knowledge of how to refer patients to internal and external resources, and the use of guidelines and protocols.
- Skills in written documentation.
- Skills in electronic documentation (including computers, telephones, fax machines, and other electronic forms of communication).

FORMS OF DOCUMENTATION

The telehealth nurse must understand and use proficiently the nursing process. The process should be **documented** in the patient record regardless of whether the patient was seen in person or attended to by telephone. Included in the patient record is the assessment of complaint(s), allergies, a history of the present illness/injury, and a medical history. The nurse's categorization of the call as urgent, nonurgent, etc. should also be documented. The plan provided by the nurse should be documented, including a referral if one is made. An evaluation of the patient's understanding and acceptance of the plan of care should also be conducted and documented. It must be remembered that the telehealth nurse may not meet every need of the patient in a single call. Rather, the telehealth nurse's focus should be to prioritize what needs to meet first. Documentation is important to evaluate and ensure that follow-up is conducted.

APPLICATION OF HIPAA STANDARDS TO TELEMEDICINE

The Health Insurance Portability and Accountability Act (HIPAA) was passed in 1996 as a measure to protect private health information of patients. Health care centers have enacted protocols to protect this information by limiting those with access to protected health information and maintaining confidentiality standards set forth by the act. The same standards apply in telemedicine, although there is an additional component of needed safety measures because the information is passing through media or telecommunications. These systems may require increased security to prevent hacking or the transmission of data into the wrong hands. Additional security systems should be in place, such as antiviral software, encryption systems, and password-protected files. Patients should be educated about the security measures being used in order to instill confidence that their personal information is protected.

Education Theory

BANDURA'S THEORY OF SOCIAL LEARNING

In the 1970s, Bandura proposed the **theory of social learning,** in which he posited that learning develops from observing, organizing, and rehearsing behavior that has been modeled. Bandura believed that people are more likely to adopt the behavior if they value the outcomes, if the outcomes have functional value, and if the person modeling the behavior is similar to the learner and is admired because of status. Behavior is the result of observation of behavioral, environmental, and cognitive interactions. There are **4 conditions required for modeling**:

- **Attention**: The degree of attention paid to modeling can depend on many variables (physical, social, and environmental).
- **Retention**: People's ability to retain models depends on symbolic coding, creating mental images, organizing thoughts, and rehearsing (mentally or physically).
- **Reproduction**: The ability to reproduce a model depends on physical and mental capabilities.
- **Motivation**: Motivation may derive from past performances, rewards, or vicarious modeling.

TRANSTHEORETICAL MODEL OF CHANGE

The Transtheoretical Model of Change puts forth concepts applicable to the process of educating patients and their family members. The **stages of the Transtheoretical Model of Change** include the following:

1. The first stage is **precontemplation**. At this point, the patient is not aware of any need for a change in the health behavior.
2. In the next stage, **contemplation**, the patient begins to realize why the change may be necessary after recognizing that the health behavior in question is unhealthy and weighing the consequences of continuing this behavior.
3. During the stage of **preparation**, the patient imagines making the change at a future time, and starts to formulate a plan to do so.
4. The **action** stage occurs when the patient makes specific modifications in health behavior and begins to note the resulting positive changes.
5. During the **maintenance** stage, the patient is able to implement the change over time by utilizing strategies to prevent a return to previously unhealthy behaviors.
6. **Termination** is the stage at which a patient has incorporated the changed behavior into daily functioning, and the patient will not resume the previous unhealthy behavior.

Kurt Lewin
Force Field Analysis

Force field analysis was designed by Kurt Lewin, a social psychologist, to analyze both the driving forces and the restraining forces for change:

- **Driving forces** instigate and promote change, such as leaders, incentives, and competition.
- **Restraining forces** resist change, such as poor attitudes, hostility, inadequate equipment, or insufficient funds.

The educator can use this force field analysis diagram to discuss variables related to a proposed change in process:

- Write the proposed change in the center column.
- Brainstorm and list driving forces and opposed restraining forces. Score the forces. (When driving and restraining forces are in balance, this is a state of equilibrium or the status quo.)
- Discuss the value of the proposed change.
- Develop a plan to diminish or eliminate restraining forces.

Lewin's Model of Change Theory

Lewin's model of change theory may be used to help some patients make decisions for change. The nurse can educate the patient about the need for change and assist with making alterations in behavior or thoughts in order to better facilitate change; however, only the patient can truly implement the change permanently. Lewin's concept of change theory involves a three-part process:

- **Unfreezing** is the part of the model in which the patient becomes open to change, sees a need for it, and removes the boundaries inhibiting change.
- The patient then makes the **actual change** according to expected outcomes and goals.
- Finally, **refreezing** is the process of maintaining the change so that it becomes a habit, and one that the patient is likely to uphold for a long period of time.

Lewin's theory also involves either driving forces or restraining forces. Driving forces are those outside measures that support the change, while restraining forces inhibit success in implementing the change.

Principles of Education

Principles of Adult Learning

Adults have a wealth of life and/or employment experiences. Their attitudes toward education may vary considerably. There are, however, some **principles of adult learning** and typical characteristics of adult learners that an instructor should consider when planning strategies for teaching parents, families, or staff.

- Practical and goal-oriented:
  - Provide overviews or summaries and examples.
  - Use collaborative discussions with problem-solving exercises.
  - Remain organized with the goal in mind.

- Self-directed:
    - Provide active involvement, asking for input.
    - Allow different options toward achieving the goal.
    - Give them responsibilities.
- Knowledgeable:
    - Show respect for their life experiences/ education.
    - Validate their knowledge and ask for feedback.
    - Relate new material to information with which they are familiar.
- Relevancy-oriented:
    - Explain how information will be applied.
    - Clearly identify objectives.
- Motivated:
    - Provide certificates of professional advancement and/or continuing education credit for staff when possible.

LEARNING STYLES

Not all people are aware of their preferred **learning style.** A range of teaching materials and methods that relate to all three major learning preferences (visual, auditory, and kinesthetic) and that are appropriate for different ages should be available. Part of assessment for teaching involves choosing the right approach based on observation and feedback. Often presenting learners with different options gives a clue to their preferred learning style. Some people have a combined learning style.

Visual learners learn best by seeing and reading:

- Provide written directions, picture guides, or demonstrate procedures. Use charts and diagrams.
- Provide photos, videos.

Auditory learners learn best by listening and talking:

- Explain procedures while demonstrating and have the learner repeat.
- Plan extra time to discuss and answer questions.
- Provide audiotapes.

Kinesthetic learners learn best by handling, doing, and practicing:

- Provide hands-on experience throughout teaching.
- Encourage handling of supplies and equipment.
- Allow the learner to demonstrate.
- Minimize instructions and allow the person to explore equipment and procedures.

BLOOM'S TAXONOMY

Bloom's taxonomy outlines behaviors that are necessary for learning and that can be applied to healthcare. The theory describes 3 types of learning.

Cognitive: Learning and gaining intellectual skills to master 6 categories of effective learning.

- Knowledge
- Comprehension
- Application
- Analysis
- Synthesis
- Evaluation

Affective: Recognizing 5 categories of feelings and values from simple to complex. This is slower to achieve than cognitive learning.

- **Receiving phenomena**: Accepting need to learn
- **Responding to phenomena**: Taking active part in care
- **Valuing**: Understanding value of becoming independent in care
- **Organizing values**: Understanding how surgery/treatment has improved life
- **Internalizing values**: Accepting condition as part of life, being consistent and self-reliant

Psychomotor: Mastering 7 categories of motor skills necessary for independence. This follows a progression from simple to complex.

- **Perception**: Uses sensory information to learn tasks
- **Set**: Shows willingness to perform tasks
- **Guided response**: Follows directions
- **Mechanism**: Does specific tasks
- **Complex overt response**: Displays competence in self-care
- **Adaptation**: Modifies procedures as needed
- **Origination**: Creatively deals with problems

APPROACHES TO TEACHING

There are many approaches to teaching, and the educator must prepare, present, and coordinate a wide range of educational workshops, lectures, discussions, and one-on-one instructions on any chosen topic. All types of classes will be needed, depending upon the purpose and material:

- **Educational workshops** are usually conducted with small groups, allowing for maximal participation. They are especially good for demonstrations and practice sessions.
- **Lectures** are often used for more academic or detailed information that may include questions and answers but limits discussion. An effective lecture should include some audiovisual support.
- **Discussions** are best with small groups so that people can actively participate. This is a good method for problem solving.
- **One-on-one instruction** is especially helpful for targeted instruction in procedures for individuals.
- **Online learning modules** are good for independent learners.

Participants should be asked to evaluate the presentations in the forms of surveys or suggestions, but ultimately the program is evaluated in terms of patient outcomes.

Teaching Techniques

There are many teaching techniques the nurse can utilize when educating patients. The nurse can demonstrate skills repeatedly when teaching and then allow the patient as much time as needed to practice the skill. The nurse should use equipment that will be available in the home and provide written instructions that can be referred to later if needed. Encouraging discussion of the information helps the patient understand and clarify. Discussion also allows the patient to vent emotions about the disease and the learning process, and to assimilate the information so that a change in behavior can result. Discussion provides feedback to the patient and encouragement to continue learning. Teaching groups of people may be appropriate when there are others who require the same information. The members can support each other with encouragement, empathy, and camaraderie, although some patients will not learn well in groups and will need individual teaching. Groups must be followed up with on an individual basis to give the chance to clarify information, to evaluate the level of learning and goal achievement, and to alter the learning plan as needed for each person.

Instruction Group Sizes

Both one-on-one instruction and group instruction have a place in patient/family education.

- **One-on-one instruction** is the most costly for an institution because it is time intensive. However, it allows the patient and family more interaction with the nurse instructor and allows them to have more control over the process by asking questions or having the instructor repeat explanations or demonstrations. One-on-one instruction is especially valuable when patients and families must learn particular skills, such as managing dialysis, or if confidentiality is important.
- **Group instruction** is the less costly because the needs of a number of people can be met at one time. Group presentations are more planned and usually scheduled for a particular time period (an hour, for example), so patients and families have less control. Questioning is usually more limited and may be done only at the end. Group instruction allows patients/families with similar health problems to interact. Group instruction is especially useful for general types of instruction, such as managing diet or other lifestyle issues.

Resources to Use When Teaching Patients and Their Families

Many hospitals that find the need to repeatedly teach the same information to patients and families prepare brochures or other written materials or teaching videos that are available for use. The nurse should review material first and make notes specific to the patient. The nurse should also watch the video with the patient and discuss it afterwards. Written materials can augment lecture and demonstrations and are useful for the patient to keep for later reference.

There are also commercial materials that can be used, provided by various drug or equipment companies. **Teaching resources** are available online from the National Institutes of Health and other reputable sources. The nurse can use these prepared materials whenever possible to save time for actual teaching but must remember to customize them to the patient. They help provide pictures, colors, and interesting features that keep the patient's interest in learning alive. There are also many books, groups, and websites that the patient should be made aware of for resources after discharge.

Readability

Studies have indicated that learning is more effective if oral presentations and/or demonstrations are supplemented with reading materials, such as handouts. **Readability** (the grade level of the material) is a concern because many patients and families may have limited English skills or low literacy, and it can be difficult for the nurse to assess people's reading level. The average American reads effectively at the 6th to 8th grade level (regardless of education achieved), but many health education materials have a much higher readability level. Additionally, research indicates that even people with much higher reading skills learn medical and health information most effectively when the material is presented at the 6th to 8th grade readability level. Therefore, patient education materials (and consent forms) should not be written at higher than 6th to 8th grade level. Readability index calculators are available on the internet to give an approximation of grade level and difficulty for those preparing materials without expertise in teaching reading.

VIDEOS

Videos are a useful adjunct to teaching as they reduce the time needed for one-on-one instruction (increasing cost-effectiveness). Passive presentation of **videos**, such as in the waiting area, has little value, but focused viewing in which the nurse discusses the purpose of the video presentation prior to viewing and then is available for discussion after viewing can be very effective. Patients and/or families are often nervous about learning patient care and are unsure of their abilities, so they may not focus completely when the nurse is presenting information. Allowing the patients/families to watch a video demonstration or explanation first and allowing them to stop or review the video presentation can help them to grasp the fundamentals before they have to apply them, relieving some of the anxiety they may be experiencing. Videos are much more effective than written materials for those with low literacy or poor English skills. The nurse should always be available to answer questions and discuss the material after the patients/families finish viewing.

LEARNING CONTRACT

In order to be compliant with a therapeutic regimen, the patient needs information about the disease, the purpose of medications and treatments, and side effects and complications to watch for. A written **learning contract** organizes this information into specific learning goals, demonstrates the importance of the information, and ensures that all pertinent information is taught. Others on the healthcare team can note patient progress and easily determine what to teach next. The patient has a written plan to follow as well.

The learning contract should take into consideration the patient's age, sex, cultural and religious values, and educational level achieved. One must consider the patient's financial status, socio-economic status, living situation, and support network. The complex nature of a therapeutic regimen combined with distracters such as side effects, pain, denial, and fear can weaken the patient's resolve to maintain compliance. One must evaluate the patient's attitudes towards healthcare, coping mechanisms, and motivation and provide reinforcement as needed.

READINESS TO LEARN

The patient/family's readiness to learn should be assessed because if they are not ready, instruction is of little value. Often readiness is indicated when the patient/family asks questions or shows and interest in procedures. There are a number of factors related to readiness to learn:

- **Physical factors:** There are a number of physical factors than can affect ability. Manual dexterity may be required to complete a task, and this varies by age and condition. Hearing or vision deficits may impact a person's ability to learn. Complex tasks may be too difficult for some because of weakness or cognitive impairment, and modifications of the environment may be needed. Health status, age, and gender may all impact the ability to learn.

- **Experience:** People's experience with learning can vary widely and is affected by their ability to cope with changes, their personal goals, motivation to learn, and cultural background. People may have widely divergent ideas about what constitutes illness and/or treatment. Lack of English skills may make learning difficult and prevent people from asking questions.
- **Mental/emotional status:** The external support system and internal motivation may impact readiness. Anxiety, fear, or depression about one's condition can make learning very difficult because the patient/family cannot focus on learning, so the nurse must spend time to reassure the patient/family and wait until they are emotionally more receptive.
- **Knowledge/education:** The knowledge base of the patient/family, their cognitive ability, and their learning styles all affect their readiness to learn. The nurse should always begin by assessing what knowledge the patient/family already has about their disease, condition, or treatment and then build form that base. People with little medical experience may lack knowledge of basic medical terminology, interfering with their ability and readiness to learn.

EDUCATIONAL GOALS, OBJECTIVES, AND PLANS

Once a topic for performance improvement education has been chosen, then goals, measurable objectives with strategies, and lesson plans must be developed. A class should stay focused on one topic rather than trying to cover many. For example:

Goal: Increase compliance with hand hygiene standards in ICU.

Objectives:

- Develop series of posters and fliers by June 1.
- Observe 100% compliance with hand hygiene standards at 2 weeks, 1-month, and 2-month intervals after training is completed.

Strategies: Conduct 4 classes at different times over a one-week period, May 25-31.

- Place posters in all nursing units, staff rooms, and utility rooms by January 3.
- Develop slide show presentation for class and provide online access to the presentation for all staff by May 25.
- Utilize handwashing kits.

Lesson plans: Discussion period: Why do we need 100% compliance?

- Slide show: The case for hand hygiene
- Discussion: What did you learn?
- Demonstration and activities to show effectiveness
- Handwashing technique

LEARNER OUTCOMES

When the quality professional plans an educational offering, whether it be a class, an online module, a workshop, or educational materials, the professional should identify **learner outcomes,** which should be conveyed to the learners from the very beginning so that they are aware of the expectations. The subject matter of the educational material and the learner outcomes should be directly related. For example, if the quality professional is giving a class on decontamination of the environment, then a learner outcome might be: "Identify the difference between disinfectants and antiseptics." There may be one or multiple learner outcomes, but part of the assessment at the end of the learning experience should be to determine if, in fact, the learner outcomes have been achieved. A survey of whether or not the learners felt that they had achieved the learner outcomes can give valuable feedback and guidance to the quality professional.

Implementation and Evaluation of Teaching Plan

Implementation and evaluation of the teaching plan includes:

- Follow teaching plan but be flexible and alter plan to suit the patient's learning needs.
- Work with a healthcare team to follow the teaching plan and ensure consistency in teaching methods as well as coordinate efforts and take responsibility for altering the plan and evaluating learning to meet goals.
- Monitor patient's motivational level, encourage with positive feedback as needed, and record patient responses to teaching and changes in behaviors as a result of all teaching sessions.
- Use tools, such as checklists, rating scales, observed behavior, written tests, and the nature of the questions from the patient when evaluating the effectiveness of the teaching plan in reaching the patient's goals for learning.
- Evaluate the plan after each session and at the end.

Communicate information taught and patient learning to any home health or community nurses involved. They can then continue the patient's teaching by evaluating behavior in the home and continuing to address learning needs as they arise.

Evaluating Effectiveness of Education

Education, like all interventions, must be evaluated for **effectiveness**. Two determinants of effectiveness include:

- **Behavior modification** involves thorough observation and measurement, identifying behavior that needs to be changed and then planning and instituting interventions to modify that behavior. The nurse can use a variety of techniques, including demonstrations of appropriate behavior, reinforcement, and monitoring until new behavior is adopted consistently. This is especially important when longstanding procedures and habits of behavior are changed.
- **Compliance rates** are often determined by observation, which should be done at intervals and on multiple occasions, but with patients, this may depend on self-reports. Outcomes is another measure of compliance; that is, if education is intended to improve patient health and reduce risk factors and that occurs, it is a good indication that there is compliance. Compliance rates are calculated by determining the number of events/procedures and degree of compliance.

Teaching Elderly Patients

The elderly patient's level of functioning must be assessed before teaching. Cognitive abilities and mental functioning may be affected by illness and aging:

- Short-term memory loss can affect the amount of material retained.
- Concentration may be decreased.
- Reaction time is delayed.
- Color discrimination, general vision, and hearing may be decreased.

The nurse should **pace** the teaching accordingly and **tailor** materials for any deficits. Family should be present for teaching if possible, to help the patient to remember key points after discharge. Large print on non-glare paper that is easy to read should be used. The nurse should use color-coding cues only if colors are easily perceived. The learning environment must be quiet and comfortable with no distractions or interruptions.

- Repeat information numerous times and allow the patient as much practice time as needed.
- Use audio-visual aids to reinforce information given verbally.
- Face the patient when speaking and encourage him/her to use hearing devices if used.
- Make sure the lighting in the room is adequate.

Teaching Patients with Learning Disabilities

Determine the type of learning disability in order to design teaching:

- When a patient has a **visual problem**, the nurse should use **verbal teaching**, repeated several times as needed and record the session for the patient to hear later if possible or use prepared audiotapes or CDs containing the information. The patient should verbalize learning to show attainment of the learning goal.
- When **auditory perception** is a problem, learning materials should be **visual** with as few words as possible. Demonstration, role-playing, and practicing the procedure will be useful to the patient. Printed materials should employ pictures, and computer use can be useful.
- If the patient has an **expressive problem**, he/she needs time to process the input and to ask questions. **Hand gestures, demonstrations, and the senses** should be utilized for teaching when appropriate.

A developmental disability will require information presented in a format that is appropriate for the person's developmental level. The nurse should keep explanations simple, and use gestures, demonstrations, activities, and repetition to teach.

Teaching to Disabled Patients and Families

The teaching of disabled patients and their families begins with an assessment of the family's willingness and preparation for the heavy duty of care that will be required. The nurse must teach information about diseases or disabilities as well as medications, procedures, diet, and physical therapies. The patients must be taught to perform ADLs as well as possible and caregivers taught how to assist when needed:

- Give patients enough information to understand and manage the disabilities and to empower them with a sense of control and coping.
- Don't overwhelm them with information.
- Plan the teaching to provide information according to learning readiness and priorities but be flexible and change the plan if needed.
- Utilize checklists of skills to help keep track of all that has been learned.
- Give praise, continued feedback, support, and empathy with every teaching session.
- Provide resources that patients and family can use after discharge and refer to home health for continuing support and teaching.

Importance of Patient's Culture in Design of Teaching Plan

The nurse must always assess the individual's cultural beliefs and values and not assume that they are the same as the culture on a whole. These beliefs determine what information the patient feels that they can pursue. Teaching that conflicts with these beliefs will be rejected. The patient's perception of health and the healthcare system must be determined because a lack of confidence in the teacher can impair motivation to learn. The nurse must **assess the patient's beliefs** about the following to develop a personalized teaching plan:

- Body image, self-esteem
- Abilities and level of knowledge
- Principles of living
- Diet, activity, health practices
- Involvement of family and support persons
- Physical and mental health and disease
- Causes of disease
- Aging
- Gender issues
- Spirituality, customs, rituals, religious precepts

Professional Practice

Scope and Standards of Practice of the Advanced Practice Nurse

ADVANCED PRACTICE REGISTERED NURSING

Advanced practice registered nursing (APRN), according to the National Council of State Boards of Nursing (NCSBN), is acting as a nurse with a foundation on **information and proficiency** that was obtained in basic nursing school. This nurse has a license to be an RN and has completed and received a diploma from graduate school in an APRN program that has been accredited from a nationwide accrediting body. This nurse has up-to-date **certification** from a nationwide certification board to work in the proper APRN specialty.

STANDARDS OF PRACTICE

Standards of practice for the APRN are defined by the ANA (from 1998) and meant to act as professional guidelines regarding the excellence of performance, service, and learning. They outline the level of work deemed satisfactory to meet the requirements of the role. These standards also provide patients with a reference to determine the quality of the treatment that was given to them. There are both **broad and particular standards** to each area of expertise. Some particular areas of expertise have their own standards as well, such as National Association of Pediatric Nursing Practitioners (NAPNP) and Association for Women's Health, Obstetric, and Neonatal Nurses (AWHONN). PNP also has separate standards. All standards may be used in legal proceedings, but they are not originally meant for this purpose.

SCOPE OF PRACTICE

The scope of practice for the APRN is dependent on each state and what the APRN in this position can do according to the Nurse Practice Act for that state. The **scope** provides **guidelines** instead of particular directives, which may be wide in range, depending on the state. Many times, the scope is founded on what is allowed legally both in the state and in the nation. The initial Scope of Practice for PNPs was created in 1983 by the National Association of Pediatric Nurse Practitioners, and has been updated multiple times since. The APRN's scope of practice is always changing and improving to meet the needs of the community, state, and country at large.

CREDENTIALS

Advanced practice registered nurses (APRN) are comprised of nurse anesthetists, nurse midwives, nurse practitioners, and clinical nurse specialists. These specialties must have proper **credentials** and take responsibility for the patient's care. Some other nurses who hold leadership responsibilities are not included under the term APRN. These nurses who are not included may have professional responsibilities but not in a clinical setting, such as teachers, administrators, or researchers, even though these nurses may have the same knowledge as an APRN. Someone that is not working in direct patient care with patients or in a family medical clinic cannot be considered an APRN.

PURPOSES OF CREDENTIALS

Purposes of credentials for the APRN are to:

- Ensure there is accountability for proficient work.
- Authenticate that the practitioner has received the correct education, has a license, and is certified.

- Ensure that the local and national laws are followed.
- Recognize the growing scope for the APRN.
- Allow an avenue for patients to make a grievance.
- Ensure a responsibility to the community by making sure standards of practice are met.

RESPONSIBILITIES

Advanced practice registered nurse (APRN) **responsibilities** include but are not limited to the following:

- Evaluate the patient, produce and assess information; comprehend complex nursing practice and practice critical thinking.
- Assess many kinds of information; compile the differential diagnosis; determine proper medical care.
- Without supervision, determine how to handle difficult patient issues.
- Create a way to identify the condition, create objectives for the patient's medical management, and stipulate the medical routine or plan.
- Plan, modify and implement the medical plan. This includes prescribing and administering drugs that fall within the APRN's scope and specialty.
- Treat the patient's physical and mental condition.
- Maintain the privacy of the patient.
- Conduct care within a therapeutic environment.

CONSULTATION, REFERRAL, AND COORDINATION

As part of the scope of practice, the advanced practice nurse is able to provide and augment primary care to patients through a number of different services:

- **Consultation** services may include a variety of services, such as assessment of growth and development and risk factors, providing interventions, such as diet and exercise programs, and educating patients.
- **Referral services** include referring patients to physicians, such as orthopedic specialists, and to organizations or agencies, such as drug rehabilitation programs.
- **Coordination services,** with the nurse maintaining contact and receiving reports from referrals in order to provide an integrated plan of care, serves as a valuable service to patients, who often must deal with many different healthcare providers who have little or no contact with each other. This type of service can prevent unnecessary duplications of service but also ensure that findings are not overlooked.

PRESCRIPTION AND DIAGNOSTICS

Both prescribing medications and treatment and ordering diagnostic tests are within the scope of practice of nurse practitioners, but as with other aspects of practice, each state establishes how that will be carried out. Additionally, insurance reimbursement varies from one area to another and must be considered:

- **Prescription:** Terminology varies from state to state with nurse practitioners allowed to "furnish" or "prescribe" some types of medications. In some states they may do so independently; in others, they must be "supervised" by a physician under whose auspices they provide care to patients. The nurse practitioner should maintain a list of medications and consider cost-effectiveness when ordering medications.

- **Diagnostics:** Nurse practitioners can order laboratory, EKG, and radiographic tests for routine screening and health assessment as well as diagnosis based on assessment. There are limitations, depending upon the individual state nursing practice act.

APRN Billing, Reimbursement, and Insurance

MEDICAL SERVICE REIMBURSEMENT FOR APRN

An advanced practice registered nurse (APRN) must be reimbursed regardless of whether the APRN works alone, has a joint practice, works in a hospital, or works in managed care. Many times, **federal policies** for Medicaid or Medicare provide this payment under fee-for-service (the APRN is paid based on claims submitted for each service that was billed) or through a Medicare Advantage Plan. Although the federal government includes directives that promote paying the medical worker (who is not a doctor) in a non-circuitous manner, it is common to find that there are **obstacles** due to state rules and regulations.

MEDICAID AND MEDICARE OBRA FOR APRNS

In 1989, the **Omnibus Budget Reconciliation Act** (OBRA) made it obligatory for there to be **Medicaid reimbursement payment** to certified children and family nurse practitioners. This started in July of 1990. The practitioner must practice within the APRN scope of practice in that state and does not require the supervision of a physician or another medical professional in these settings. The amount to be paid is contingent upon the state, but is in the range of 70%–100% of the fee-for-service physician fee outlined by Medicaid. Children and family nurse practitioners are allowed to send an invoice directly to Medicaid in a non-circuitous manner after getting a provider number from the Medicaid agency for the particular state. Each state can legalize expanding Medicaid reimbursement to additional types of APRNs that are not listed in the federal mandates, such as certified registered nurse anesthetists.

If the APRN conducts **"incident to"** work (work conducted by an APRN under the supervision of a physician), the invoice is given to Medicare/Medicaid by the doctor that has hired the APRN, and it has to be in the doctor's name with that provider number and CPT code. This will be paid with a total physician fee and the money comes to the doctor or to the doctor's practice.

MALPRACTICE INSURANCE

Malpractice insurance will not shield an APRN from being **liable** for giving medical attention with **no license to do so** in a case where the APRN is acting beyond what he or she is legally allowed to do in the particular state. The **National Practitioner Data Bank** gathers data regarding actions in opposition to medical professionals. Nurses are included in the data bank. Malpractice insurance may be occurrence coverage or claims-made coverage, with optional tail coverage.

- **Occurrence coverage** is for an instance that happened when the policy was in effect, even if the date of discovery or the claim was filed after a point when the coverage ended.
- **Claims-made coverage** is for claims made inside the time that the policy was in effect, even if the instance happened at another time.
- **Optional tail coverage** makes the coverage go even further on a claims-made policy so that any subsequent claims that may come up as time goes by are covered even if the basic claims-made coverage time is over.

Ethics

ETHICAL PRINCIPLES

Autonomy is the ethical principle that the individual has the right to make decisions about his or her own care. In the case of children or patients with dementia who cannot make autonomous decisions, parents or family members may serve as the legal decision maker. The nurse must keep the patient and/or family fully informed so that they can exercise their autonomy in informed decision-making.

Justice is the ethical principle that relates to the distribution of the limited resources of healthcare benefits to the members of society. These resources must be distributed fairly. This issue may arise if there is only one bed left and two sick patients. Justice comes into play in deciding which patient should stay and which should be transported or otherwise cared for. The decision should be made according to what is best or most just for the patients and not colored by personal bias.

Beneficence is an ethical principle that involves performing actions that are for the purpose of benefitting another person. In the care of a patient, any procedure or treatment should be done with the ultimate goal of benefitting the patient, and any actions that are not beneficial should be reconsidered. As conditions change, procedures need to be continually reevaluated to determine if they are still of benefit.

Nonmaleficence is an ethical principle that means healthcare workers should provide care in a manner that does not cause direct intentional harm to the patient:

- The actual act must be good or morally neutral.
- The intent must be only for a good effect.
- A bad effect cannot serve as the means to get to a good effect.
- A good effect must have more benefit than a bad effect has harm.

BIOETHICS

Bioethics is a branch of ethics that involves making sure that the medical treatment given is the most morally correct choice given the different options that might be available and the differences inherent in the varied levels of treatment. In the health care unit, if the patients, family members, and the staff are in agreement when it comes to values and decision-making, then no ethical dilemma exists; however, when there is a difference in value beliefs between the patients/family members and the staff, there is a bioethical dilemma that must be resolved. Sometimes, discussion and explanation can resolve differences, but at times the institution's ethics committee must be brought in to resolve the conflict. The primary goal of bioethics is to determine the most morally correct action using the set of circumstances given.

NURSING CODE OF ETHICS

There is more interest in the **ethics** involved in healthcare due to technological advances that have made the prolongation of life, organ transplants, prenatal manipulation, and saving of premature infants possible, sometimes with poor outcomes. Couple these with healthcare's limited resources, and **ethical dilemmas** abound. Ethics is the study of **morality** as the value that controls actions. The American Nurses Association Code of Ethics contains nine statements defining **principles** the nurse can use when faced with moral and ethical problems. Nurses must be knowledgeable about the many ethical issues in healthcare and about the field of ethics in general. The nurse must help a patient to reveal their values and morals to the health care team so that the patient, family, and team can resolve moral issues pertaining to the patient's care. As part of the healthcare team, the nurse has a right to express personal values and moral concerns about medical issues.

Ethical Decision-Making Model

There are many ethical decision-making models. Some general guidelines to apply in using ethical decision-making models could be the following:

- Gather information about the identified problem
- State reasonable alternatives and solutions to the problem
- Utilize ethical resources (for example, clergy or ethics committees) to help determine the ethically important elements of each solution or alternative
- Suggest and attempt possible solutions
- Choose a solution to the problem

It is important to always consider the **ethical principles** of autonomy, beneficence, nonmaleficence, justice, and fidelity when attempting to facilitate ethical decision-making with family members, caregivers, and the healthcare team.

Ethical Assessment

While the terms *ethics* and *morals* are sometimes used interchangeably, ethics is a study of morals and encompasses concepts of right and wrong. When making **ethical assessments,** one must consider not only what people should do but also what they actually do, as these two things are sometimes at odds. Ethical issues can be difficult to assess because of personal bias, which is one of the reasons that sharing concerns with other internal sources and reaching consensus is so valuable. Issues of concern might include options for care, refusal of care, rights to privacy, adequate relief of suffering, and the right to self-determination. Internal sources might include the ethics committee, whose role is to make decisions regarding ethical issues. Risk management can provide guidance related to personal and institutional liability. External agencies might include government agencies, such as the public health department.

Ethical Analysis of a Situation

Assessment of the situation is done to reveal the **ethical, legal, and professional conflicts** that are present. Those who are involved are identified, including the patient, family, and healthcare personnel. The decision maker is determined if it is not the patient. Information about the situation is collected to determine medical facts about the disease and condition of the patient, options for treatment, and nursing diagnoses. Any pertinent legal information is included. The patient and family's cultural, religious, and moral values are determined. Possible courses of action are listed and compared in terms of outcomes for the patient using the utilitarian or deontological theory of ethics. Professional codes of ethics are also applied. A decision is made and evaluated as to whether it is the most morally correct action. Ethical arguments for and against the decision are given and responded to by the decision maker.

Professional Boundaries

Gifts

Over time, patients may develop a bond with nurses they trust and may feel grateful to the nurse for the care provided and want to express thanks, but the nurse must make sure to maintain professional boundaries. Patients often offer **gifts** to nurses to show their appreciation, but some adults, especially those who are weak and ill or have cognitive impairment, may be taken advantage of easily. Patients may offer valuables and may sometimes be easily manipulated into giving large sums of money. Small tokens of appreciation that can be shared with other staff, such as a box of chocolates, are usually acceptable (depending upon the policy of the institution), but almost any other gifts (jewelry, money, clothes) should be declined: "I'm sorry, that's so kind of you, but nurses are not allowed to accept gifts from patients." Declining may relieve the patient of the feeling of obligation.

SEXUAL RELATIONS

When the boundary between the role of the professional nurse and the vulnerability of the patient is breached, a boundary violation occurs. Because the nurse is in the position of authority, the responsibility to maintain the boundary rests with the nurse; however, the line separating them is a continuum and sometimes not easily defined. It is inappropriate for nurses to engage in **sexual relations** with patients, and if the sexual behavior is coerced or the patient is cognitively impaired, it is **illegal**. However, more common violations with adults, particularly elderly patients, include exposing a patient unnecessarily, using sexually demeaning gestures or language (including off-color jokes), harassment, or inappropriate touching. Touching should be used with care, such as touching a hand or shoulder. Hugging may be misconstrued.

ATTENTION

Nursing is a giving profession, but the nurse must temper giving with recognition of professional boundaries. Patients have many needs. As acts of kindness, nurses (especially those involved in home care) often give certain patients extra attention and may offer to do **favors**, such as cooking or shopping. They may become overly invested in the patients' lives. While this may benefit a patient in the short term, it can establish a relationship of increasing **dependency** and **obligation** that does not resolve the long-term needs of the patient. Making referrals to the appropriate agencies or collaborating with family to find ways to provide services is more effective. Becoming overly invested may be evident by the nurse showing favoritism or spending too much time with the patient while neglecting other duties. On the other end of the spectrum are nurses who are disinterested and fail to provide adequate attention to the patient's detriment. Lack of adequate attention may lead to outright neglect.

COERCION

Power issues are inherent in matters associated with professional boundaries. Physical abuse is both unprofessional and illegal, but behavior can easily border on abusive without the patient being physically injured. Nurses can easily **intimidate** older adults and sick patients into having procedures or treatments they do not want. Regardless of age, patients have the right to choose and the right to refuse treatment. Difficulties arise with cognitive impairment, and in that case, another responsible adult (often the patient's child or spouse) is designated to make decisions, but every effort should be made to gain patient cooperation. Forcing the patient to do something against his or her will borders on abuse and can sometimes degenerate into actual abuse if physical coercion is involved.

PERSONAL INFORMATION

When pre-existing personal or business relationships exist, other nurses should be assigned care of the patient whenever possible, but this may be difficult in small communities. However, the nurse should strive to maintain a professional role separate from the personal role and respect professional boundaries. The nurse must respect and maintain the confidentiality of the patient and family members, but the nurse must also be very careful about **disclosing personal information** about him or herself because this establishes a social relationship that interferes with the professional role of the nurse and the boundary between the patient and the nurse. The nurse and patient should never share secrets. When the nurse divulges personal information, he or she may become vulnerable to the patient, a reversal of roles.

Patient Rights

PATIENT RIGHTS AND RESPONSIBILITIES

Empowering patients and families to act as their own advocates requires they have a clear understanding of their **rights and responsibilities.** These should be given (in print form) and/or presented (audio/video) to patients and families on admission or as soon as possible:

- **Rights** should include competent, non-discriminatory medical care that respects privacy and allows participation in decisions about care and the right to refuse care. They should have clear understandable explanations of treatments, options, and conditions, including outcomes. They should be apprised of transfers, changes in care plan, and advance directives. They should have access to medical records information about charges.
- **Responsibilities** should include providing honest and thorough information about health issues and medical history. They should ask for clarification if they don't understand information that is provided to them, and they should follow the plan of care that is outlined or explain why that is not possible. They should treat staff and other patients with respect.

INFORMED CONSENT

Patients or guardians must provide informed consent for all treatment the patient receives. This includes a thorough explanation of all procedures and treatment and associated risks. Patients/guardians should be apprised of all options and allowed input on the type of treatments. Patients/guardians should be apprised of all reasonable risks and any complications that might be life threatening or increase morbidity. The American Medical Association has established **guidelines for informed consent:**

- Explanation of diagnosis
- Nature and reason for treatment or procedure
- Risks and benefits
- Alternative options (regardless of cost or insurance coverage)
- Risks and benefits of alternative options
- Risks and benefits of not having a treatment or procedure
- Providing informed consent is a requirement of all states

Note: A patient may waive their right to informed consent; if this is the case, the nurse should document the patient's refusal and proceed with the procedure. Also, informed consent is not necessary for procedures performed to save a life/limb in which the patient/family is unable to consent.

CONFIDENTIALITY

Confidentiality is the obligation that is present in a professional-patient relationship. Nurses are under an obligation to protect the information they possess concerning the patient and family. Care should be taken to safeguard that information and provide the privacy that the family deserves. This is accomplished through the use of required passwords when family call for information about the patient and through the limitation of who is allowed to visit. There may be times when confidentiality must be broken to save the life of a patient, but those circumstances are rare. The nurse must make all efforts to safeguard patient records and identification. Computerized record keeping should be done in such a way that the screen is not visible to others, and paper records must be secured.

Legal Regulations

ADVANCE DIRECTIVES

In accordance to Federal and state laws, individuals have the right to self-determination in health care, including the right to make decisions about end of life care through **advance directives** such as living wills and the right to assign a surrogate person to make decisions through a durable power of attorney. Patients should routinely be questioned about an advanced directive as they may present at a healthcare provider without the document. Patients who have indicated that they desire a do-not-resuscitate (DNR) order should not receive resuscitative treatments for terminal illness or conditions in which meaningful recovery cannot occur. Patients and families of those with terminal illnesses should be questioned as to whether the patients are Hospice patients. For those with DNR requests or those withdrawing life support, staff should provide the patient palliative rather than curative measures, such as pain control and/or oxygen, and emotional support to the patient and family. Religious traditions and beliefs about death should be treated with respect.

REGULATION OF NURSING BY STATES' NURSE PRACTICE ACT

Each state's **nurse practice act** seeks to regulate nursing within the state. It specifies the amount and type of education required to become an **RN**. It defines the RN's role and responsibilities in healthcare settings. It lists actions that the nurse may take and defines advanced practice education, experience, responsibilities, and limitations. It gives nurses the authorization to perform as required. It also regulates delegation and supervision responsibilities of the nurse. Nurse practice acts are administered by the state board of nursing, which is responsible for issuing and renewing nurse licenses as well as discipline and censure of nurses. Most state boards of nursing now have a website that provides state-specific information about licensure and nursing rights and responsibilities.

NURSE'S ACCOUNTABILITY FOR NURSING CARE

Nurses are part of an interdisciplinary team responsible for patient outcomes. Nurses have the responsibility for the outcomes of nursing care as a professional group. This responsibility is outlined in each state's nurse practice act, the American Nurses Association (ANA) practice guidelines, and the nurse's job description. Tools, such as the nursing care plan that includes standardized nursing diagnoses, interventions, and expected outcomes, enable the nurse to fulfill this responsibility. Empowerment to act as the patient advocate allows the nurse to point out factors in the patient's individual situation that can be addressed to further improve outcome. Critical thinking during decision-making and detailed documentation are also important. The nurse is held accountable for delegation as well as supervising care by others and evaluation of the outcomes of that care as well. The nurse has personal **accountability** in terms of ethical and moral conduct. Since clinical knowledge is crucial to critical thinking, the nurse must strive to increase knowledge continuously through professional development throughout his or her career.

HIPAA

The Health Insurance Portability and Accountability Act (HIPAA) and state laws govern **who may receive healthcare information** about a person, how permission is to be obtained, how the information may be shared, and patients' rights concerning personal information. HIPAA strives to protect the **privacy** of an individual's healthcare information. Facilities must prevent this information from being accessed by unauthorized personnel. Healthcare information is required to be protected on the **administrative**, **physical**, and **technical** levels. The patient must sign a release form to allow any sharing of patient information. There are stiff penalties for violation of these laws, ranging from $100 for an unintentional violation to $50,000 for a willful violation. Facilities that violate HIPAA may also be subject to corrective actions. Penalties are governed by the Department of Health and Human Services' Office for Civil Right and the state attorneys general.

APPLICATION OF HIPAA TO PRACTICE

As an integral member of the health care team, the nurse must always be aware of HIPAA regulations and apply this knowledge to practice. The nurse is responsible for the following efforts to protect and maintain patient privacy:

- The nurse must read and follow facility policies regarding the transfer of patient data.
- Communication between health care personnel about a patient should always be in a private place so that this information is not overheard by those who do not have the right to share the information.
- Access to charts must be restricted to only those health care team members involved in that patient's care.
- Patient care information for unlicensed workers cannot be posted at the bedside, but must be on a care plan or the patient chart in a protected area.
- The nurse must not give information casually to anyone (e.g., visitors or family members) unless it is confirmed that they have the right to have that information.
- Family members must not be relied upon to interpret for the patient; an interpreter must be obtained to protect patient privacy.
- Computers with patient information must have passwords and safeguards to prevent unauthorized access of patient information.
- The nurse should not leave voicemail messages containing protected healthcare information for a patient but should instead ask the patient to call back.

> **Review Video: What is HIPAA?**
> Visit mometrix.com/academy and enter code: 412009

OSHA

The **Occupational Safety and Health Act (OSHA)** seeks to keep workers safe and healthy while on the job. OSHA mandates that employers maintain a safe environment, workers are made fully aware of any hazards, and that access to personal protective gear is made available to workers who come into contact with hazardous materials. By following these regulations, an employer keeps injury and illness of workers to an absolute minimum. This fosters productivity, since workers are not absent due to illness or injury, employee health costs are contained, and the turnover rate is decreased, saving money spent on hiring and training new employees. OSHA is concerned about healthcare employee exposure to radiation, as well as chemical and biological agents, when caring for patients. Information is available to help hospitals and other facilities write plans that comply with best practices to deal with this and other threats to employees. Cleaning procedures, decontamination, and hazardous waste disposal are all covered by OSHA and apply to everyday hospital operation as well as disaster situations.

> **Review Video: What is OSHA (Occupational Safety and Health Administration)**
> Visit mometrix.com/academy and enter code: 913559

AHRQ

The **Agency for Healthcare Research and Quality (AHRQ)** is part of the U.S. Department of Health and Human Services. This agency is concerned about health care and primarily promotes scientific research into the safety, effectiveness, and quality of healthcare. It encourages evidence-based healthcare that produces the best possible outcome while containing healthcare costs. It makes contracts with institutions to review any published evidence on healthcare in order to produce reports used by other organizations to write guidelines. The agency operates the National Guideline Clearinghouse, which is available online. It is a repository of evidence-based guidelines that address various health conditions and diseases. These guidelines are written by many different health-related professional organizations and are used by primary healthcare providers, nurses, and healthcare facilities to guide patient treatment and care.

OBRA 1987

The **Omnibus Budget Reconciliation Act of 1987 (OBRA 1987)**, also known as the Nursing Home Reform Act, instituted requirements for nursing homes with the purpose of strengthening and protecting patient rights. These requirements are as follows: "a facility must provide each patient with a level of care that enables him or her to attain or maintain the highest practicable physical, mental, and psychosocial wellbeing." OBRA 1987 required that all nursing home patients receive an initial evaluation with yearly follow-ups. Every patient is required to have a comprehensive care plan. Patients were ensured the right to medical care and the right to be informed about and refuse medical treatment. OBRA 1987 requires each state to establish, monitor, and enforce its own licensing requirements in addition to federal standards. Each state is also required to fund, staff, and maintain investigative and Ombudsman units.

OBRA 1990 (PSDA)

The Omnibus Budget Reconciliation Act of 1990 included the amendment called the **Patient Self Determination Act (PSDA)**. The PSDA required healthcare facilities to provide written information about advanced healthcare directives and the right to accept or reject medical or surgical treatments to all patients. Patients who make an advanced directive are leaving instructions about what medical interventions they authorize or refuse if they are incapacitated by illness or injury. They can also nominate another person to make these decisions for them in this situation. The PSDA also protected the right of patients to accept or refuse medical treatments. Healthcare facilities and hospitals are legally required to communicate these rights to all patients, to respect these rights, and to educate staff and personnel about these rights.

EMTALA

The **Emergency Medical Treatment and Active Labor Act (EMTALA)** is designed to prevent patient "dumping" from emergency departments (ED) and is an issue of concern for risk management that requires staff training for compliance:

- Transfers from the ED may be intrahospital or to another facility.
- Stabilization of the patient with emergency conditions or active labor must be done in the ED prior to transfer, and initial screening must be given prior to inquiring about insurance or ability to pay.
- Stabilization requires treatment for emergency conditions and reasonable belief that, although the emergency condition may not be completely resolved, the patient's condition will not deteriorate during transfer.
- Women in the ED in active labor should deliver both the child and placenta before transfer.
- The receiving department or facility should be capable of treating the patient and dealing with complications that might occur.
- Transfer to another facility is indicated if the patient requires specialized services not available intrahospital, such as to burn centers.

CMS

The **Centers for Medicare and Medicaid (CMS)**, part of the U.S. Department of Health and Human Service department, see to it that healthcare regulations are observed by healthcare facilities that receive federal reimbursement. They reimburse facilities for care given to Medicare, Medicaid, and the state Children's Health Insurance Program (CHIP) recipients. They also monitor adherence to HIPAA regulations concerning healthcare information portability and confidentiality. CMS examines documentation of patient care when deciding to reimburse for care given. CMS has regulations for all types of medical facilities, and these regulations have profoundly impacted nursing practice because nurses must ensure that they comply with regulations related to the quality of patient care and concerns regarding cost-containment. Each facility should provide guidelines to assist nursing staff in meeting the specific documentation requirements of CMS.

Abuse and Neglect

INDICATORS OF ABUSE THAT MAY BE IDENTIFIED IN THE PATIENT HISTORY

The nurse should always be aware of the presence of any **indicators** that may present a potential for or an actual situation that involves **abuse**. These indicators may present in the **patient's history**. Some examples of indicators concerning their primary complaint may include the following: vague description about the cause of the problem, inconsistencies between physical findings and explanations, minimizing injuries, long period of time between injury and treatment, and over-reactions or under-reactions of family members to injuries. Other important information may be revealed in the family genome, such as family history of violence, time spent in jail or prison, and family history of violent deaths or substance abuse. The patient's health history may include previous injuries, spontaneous abortions, or history of pervious inpatient psychiatric treatment or substance abuse.

During the collection of the patient history, the financial history, the patient's family values, and the patient's relationships with family members can also reveal actual or potential **abuse indicators**.

- The **financial history** may indicate that the patient has little or no money or that they are not given access to money by a controlling family member. They may also be unemployed or utilizing an elderly family member's income for their own personal expenses.
- **Family values** may indicate strong beliefs in physical punishment, dictatorship within the home, inability to allow different opinions within the home, or lack of trust for anyone outside the family.
- **Relationships** within the family may be dysfunctional. Problems such as lack of affection between family members, co-dependency, frequent arguments, extramarital affairs, or extremely rigid beliefs about roles within the family may be present.

During the collection of the patient history, the sexual, social, and psychological history of the patient should be evaluated for any signs of actual or potential abuse.

- The **sexual history** may reveal problems such as previous sexual abuse, forced sexual acts, sexually transmitted diseases, sexual knowledge beyond normal age-appropriate knowledge, or promiscuity.
- The **social history** may reveal unplanned pregnancies, social isolation as evidenced by lack of friends available to help the patient, unreasonable jealousy of significant other, verbal aggression, belief in physical punishment, or problems in school.

- During the **psychological assessment** the patient may express feelings of helplessness and being trapped. The patient may be unable to describe their future, become tearful, perform self-mutilation, have low self-esteem, and have had previous suicide attempts.

Nursing Observations That May Indicate Abuse

During the nursing assessment, observations may also be made by the nurse that can provide vital information about actual or potential abuse. **General observations** may include finding that the patient history is far different from what is objectively viewed by the nurse or that there is a lack of proper clothing or lack of physical care provided. The home environment may include lack of heat, water, or food. It may also reveal inappropriate sleeping arrangements or lack of an environmentally safe housing situation. Observations concerning **family communications** may reveal that the abuser answers all the questions for the whole family or that others look to the controlling member for approval or seem fearful of others. Family members may frequently argue, interrupt each other, or act out negative nonverbal behaviors while others are speaking. They may avoid talking about certain subjects that they feel are secretive.

Indicators of Abuse That May Be Evident During the Physical Assessment

During the **physical assessment** the nurse should always be aware of any **indicators of abuse**. These indicators may include increased anxiety about being examined or in the presence of the abuser; poor hygiene; looks to abuser to answer questions for them; flinching; over or underweight; presence of bruises, welts, scars or cigarette burns; bald patches on scalp for pulling out of hair; intracranial bleeding; subconjunctival hemorrhages; black eye(s); hearing loss from untreated infection or injury; poor dental hygiene; abdominal injuries; fractures; developmental delays; hyperactive reflexes; genital lacerations or ecchymosis; and presence of sexually transmitted diseases, rectal bruising, bleeding, edema, or poor sphincter tone.

Domestic Violence

Men, women, elderly, children, and the disabled may all be victims of **domestic violence**. The violent person harms physically or sexually and uses threats and fear to maintain control of the victim. The violence does not improve unless the abuser gets intensive counseling. The abuser may promise not to do it again, but the violence usually gets more frequent and worsens over time. The nurse should ask all patients in private about abuse, neglect, and fear of a caretaker. If abuse is suspected or there are signs present, the state may require **reporting**:

- Give victims information about community hotlines, shelters, and resources.
- Urge them to set up a plan for escape for themselves and any children, complete with supplies in a location away from the home.
- Assure victims that they are not at fault and do not deserve the abuse.
- Try to empower them by helping them to realize that they do not have to take abuse and can find support to change the situation.

Assessment of Domestic Violence

According to the guidelines of the Family Violence Prevention Fund, **assessment** for domestic violence should be done for all adolescent and adult patients, regardless of background or signs of abuse. While females are the most common victims, there are increasing reports of male victims of domestic violence, both in heterosexual and homosexual relationships. The person doing the assessment should be informed about domestic violence and be aware of risk factors and danger signs. The interview should be conducted in private (special accommodations may need to be made for children <3 years old). The nurse manager's office, bathrooms, and examining rooms should have information about domestic violence posted prominently. Brochures and information should be available to give to patients. Patients may present with a variety of physical complaints, such as headache, pain, palpitations, numbness, or pelvic pain. They are often depressed and may appear suicidal and may be isolated from friends and family. Victims of domestic violence often exhibit fear of spouse/partner, and may report injury inconsistent with symptoms.

STEPS TO IDENTIFYING VICTIMS OF DOMESTIC VIOLENCE

The **Family Violence Prevention Fund** has issued guidelines for identifying and assisting victims of domestic violence. There are 7 steps:

1. **Inquiry:** Non-judgmental questioning should begin with asking if the person has ever been abused—physically, sexually, or psychologically.
2. **Interview:** The person may exhibit signs of anxiety or fear and may blame himself or report that others believe he is abused. The person should be questioned if she is afraid for her life or for her children.
3. **Question:** If the person reports abuse, it's critical to ask if the person is in immediate danger or if the abuser is on the premises. The interviewer should ask if the person has been threatened. The history and pattern of abuse should be questioned, and if children are involved, whether the children are abused. Note: State laws vary, and in some states, it is mandatory to report if a child was present during an act of domestic violence as this is considered child abuse. The nurse must be aware of state laws regarding domestic and child abuse, and all nurses are mandatory reporters.
4. **Validate:** The interviewer should offer support and reassurance in a non-judgmental manner, telling the patient the abuse is not his or her fault.
5. **Give information:** While discussing facts about domestic violence and the tendency to escalate, the interviewer should provide brochures and information about safety planning. If the patient wants to file a complaint with the police, the interviewer should assist the person to place the call.
6. **Make referrals:** Information about state, local, and national organizations should be provided along with telephone numbers and contact numbers for domestic violence shelters.
7. **Document:** Record keeping should be legal, legible, and lengthy with a complete report and description of any traumatic injuries resulting from domestic violence. A body map may be used to indicate sites of injury, especially if there are multiple bruises or injuries.

INJURIES CONSISTENT WITH DOMESTIC VIOLENCE

There are a number of characteristic **injuries** that may indicate domestic violence, including ruptured eardrum; rectal/genital injury (burns, bites, or trauma); scrapes and bruises about the neck, face, head, trunk, arms; and cuts, bruises, and fractures of the face. The pattern of injuries associated with domestic violence is also often distinctive. The bathing-suit pattern involves injuries on parts of body that are usually covered with clothing as the perpetrator inflicts damage but hides evidence of abuse. Head and neck injuries (50%) are also common. Abusive injuries (rarely attributable to accidents) are common and include bites, bruises, rope and cigarette burns, and welts in the outline of weapons (belt marks). Bilateral injuries of arms/legs are often seen with domestic abuse. Defensive injuries are indicative of abuse.

Defensive injuries to the back of the body are often incurred as the victim crouches on the floor face down while being attacked. The soles of the feet may be injured from kicking at perpetrator. The ulnar aspect of hand or palm may be injured from blocking blows.

Elder Abuse

Active abuse is intentional (such as hitting) while passive abuse occurs without intention. **Elder abuse** may be difficult to diagnose, especially if the person is cognitively impaired, but symptoms can include fearfulness, disparities in reports of injuries between patient and caregiver, evidence of old or repeated injuries, poor hygiene and dental care, decubiti, malnutrition, undue concern with costs on caregiver's part, unsupportive attitude of caregiver, and caregiver's reluctance or refusal to allow patient to communicate privately with the nurse. Diagnosis includes a careful history and physical exam, including direct questioning of the patient about abuse. Treatment includes attending to injuries or physical needs, (this can vary widely) and referral to adult protective services as indicated. Reporting laws regarding elder abuse vary somewhat from one state to another, but all states have laws regarding elder abuse and most states require mandatory reporting to adult protective services by health workers.

Elder Neglect

Neglect of basic needs is a common problem of older adults who live alone or with reluctant or incapable caregivers. In some cases, passive neglect may occur because an elderly spouse is trying to take care of a patient and is unable to provide the care needed, but in other cases, active neglect reflects a lack of caring and may border on negligence and abuse. **Indications** of neglect include the following:

- Lack of assistive devices, such as cane or walker, needed for mobility
- Misplaced or missing glasses or hearing aids
- Poor dental hygiene and dental care and/or missing dentures
- Patient left unattended for extended periods of time, sometimes confined to a bed or chair
- Patient left in soiled or urine/feces-stained clothing
- Inadequate food/fluid/nutrition resulting in weight loss
- Inappropriate and unkempt clothing, such as lack of sweater or coat during the winter and dirty or torn clothing
- Dirty, messy environment

Risk of Elder Abuse

Age and disability increase the **risks of elder abuse**. People over the age of 80 are more than twice as likely to suffer abuse as younger adults. Patients with dementia, such as Alzheimer's disease, are at risk of abuse in both the home environment, where they are often cared for by adult children, and in institutions. Caregivers often lose patience and become frustrated, especially if the patient's behavior is belligerent, combative, or disruptive. This type of abuse can be very difficult to diagnose, as the patient is usually unable to corroborate abuse. In fact, even older adults who are not cognitively impaired may be afraid to report abuse because they depend on the abusers to care for them. Older adults who are dependent on others for assistance with ADLs, such as dressing, bathing, and food preparation are also particularly at risk for outright abuse and neglect. Abusers often suffer from depression and or substance abuse and may be financially dependent on the victim.

Physical and Emotional Abuse

There are a number of different types of elder abuse. **Physical abuse** is an active form of abuse and is almost always associated with **psychological abuse** as well. Older adults, particularly those cared for by family members (often an adult child) or other caregivers, may suffer various types of assaults related to hitting, kicking, pulling hair, shoving, and pushing. Caregivers may make frequent threats to hit the older adult, sometimes brandishing a weapon, if the person doesn't cooperate and may tell the person to commit suicide. Ongoing intimidation may make the patient terrified and anxious. Sometimes, caregivers threaten to injure pets or family members, increasing patient's fear. Patients may be forcibly confined, forced into seclusion, and/or force-fed to the point that they choke on food.

Physical symptoms include the following:

- Ruptured eardrum
- Rectal/genital injury—burns, bites, trauma
- Scrapes and bruises about the neck, face, head, trunk, arms
- Cuts, bruises, and fractures of the face

The **pattern of injuries** is also often distinctive:

- Bathing suit pattern—injuries on parts of body that are usually covered with clothing as the perpetrator abuses but hides evidence of abuse
- Head and neck injuries (50%)

Abusive injuries (rarely attributable to accidents) are common:

- Bites, bruises, rope and cigarette burns, welts in the outline of weapons (belt marks)
- Bilateral injuries of arms/legs

Defensive injuries are indicative of abuse:

- Back of the body injury from being attacked while crouched on the floor face down
- Soles of the feet from kicking at perpetrator
- Ulnar aspect of hand or palm from blocking blows

Psychological symptoms include anxiety, paranoia, insomnia, low self-esteem, avoidance of eye contact, and obvious nervousness in the presence of the caregiver, who is often reluctant to leave the patient alone.

SEXUAL ABUSE

Sexual abuse of older adults occurs when the person receiving sexual attention is unwilling to participate or unable (because of cognizant impairment or other illness) to consent to sexual intimacy. Types of **sexual abuse** include:

- **Physical**: Fondling, kissing, and rape
- **Emotional**: Exhibitionism
- **Verbal**: Sexual harassment, using obscene language, threatening

Sexual abuse of older adults occurs most commonly to women in their 70s or 80s confined to nursing homes. Sexual abuse may also occur in home environments, but it is harder to detect. Most abusers are fellow nursing home residents (males over the age of 60), and the most common form of abuse is sexualized kissing and fondling of genitals. Because older adults have a right to sexual intimacy, in some cases what may appear to be abuse between residents may, in fact, be consensual. Caregivers may have raped or otherwise sexually abused patients, and this exercise of power over another person is always illegal abuse.

Financial Abuse

Elder abuse often occurs when an older adult is unable to care for or protect himself. In many situations, another person takes advantage of an older adult and uses threats or manipulation to justify the activity. As older adults become unable to manage their own financial affairs, they become increasingly vulnerable to **financial abuse**, especially if they have cognitive impairment or physical impairments that impair their mobility. This kind of abuse often occurs when an older adult trusts another person for help with finances and is taken advantage of. Financial abuse includes the following:

- Outright stealing of property or persuading patients to give away possessions
- Forcing patients to sign away property
- Emptying bank and savings accounts
- Using stolen credit cards
- Convincing the person to invest money in fraudulent schemes
- Taking money for home renovations that are not done

Indications of financial abuse may be unpaid bills, unusual activity at ATMs or with credit cards, inadequate funds to meet needs, disappearance of items in the home, change in the provision of a will, and deferring to caregivers regarding financial affairs. Family or caregivers may move permanently into the patient's home and take over without sharing costs.

Some examples of financial abuse of an elderly client include when another person steals money or other valuable items, forges the patient's signature on checks or signs over Social Security income, uses the adult's name and identifying information to gain access to other accounts or to spend money, advises an older adult to invest money into accounts or schemes that are not legitimate, or commits fraud by telling an older adult that she has won money or is contributing to fraudulent organizations.

Socioeconomic Factors That May Contribute to Elder Abuse

Elder abuse is a problem that remains largely underreported. Elder abuse may be more prevalent when abusers see older adults as helpless victims who have no control over their environment or who have no access to reporting to authorities. Some older adults and their abusers may downplay the abuse or neglect, while others may be unsure of what their options are for help and safety. There are some **socioeconomic factors** that contribute to elder abuse and neglect, allowing these situations to continue. Some examples include a stressful environment, such as a long-term-care facility that houses many high-need residents, family or caregivers that are burdened by stress or who have emotional instability, the prevalence of ageism and the idea that the elderly are incompetent or frail, the increase in diagnosed cases of chronic disease, and advances in medicine and technology that allow older persons to live longer.

Screening Questions to Assess for Elder Abuse

The nurse who cares for older adults is in a position to detect cases of abuse or neglect that may otherwise go unreported. The nurse serves as the patient's advocate to protect him from abuse taking place that he may be powerless to control. The nurse may need to ask questions when the potential abuser is not in the room. Some questions that the nurse may ask to assess for underlying abuse or neglect include:

- Has anyone been hurting you?
- Do you feel safe where you live?
- Is there someone in your family/neighborhood that you are afraid of?
- Have you ever been threatened?
- Has anyone ever touched you in a manner that made you uncomfortable?
- Do you feel that your caregiver/family/friend is there for you when you need him or her?

UNDERREPORTING OF ABUSE IN LONG-TERM-CARE FACILITIES

Abusive and neglectful situations that occur in nursing homes may go **underreported** for various reasons. Many longterm-care facilities care for a large number of residents, caregivers may be stressed, and units may be understaffed. These facilities provide care for high-need patients, potentially causing difficulties with time management and fully meeting the needs of every resident, which further contributes to abuse. Some residents may be in situations where they are unable to report any abuse because of speech or hearing difficulties, physical disabilities, or cognitive changes. Abuse or neglect may also occur and remain underreported in residents who do not have regular visits from families or friends. These residents may go for long periods without an outside person visiting to evaluate or notice any changes in behavior or appearance that may occur with abuse.

Health Promotion and Disease Prevention

BENEFITS OF KNOWING EPIDEMIOLOGICAL PRACTICES

Epidemiology is important to nurses across all clinical settings, not just those in public health positions. Each and every nurse will treat a varied patient population during his or her career, and it is important for the nurse to create a plan of care that is tailored to the patient; the patient's age, race, career, and religion all represent different populations to which he or she belongs, and may affect clinical course, treatment, and outcome. Armed with **epidemiological knowledge** about his or her patients, the nurse can create a clinical decision-making framework, an effective care plan, and the means to share this information with his or her peers to aid in the care of other patients.

HEALTH PROMOTION

Nurses promote health when they assist individuals to change behavior in ways that help them to attain and maintain the highest level of wellbeing possible. Health promotion is a very popular way to control healthcare costs and reduce illness and early death. Health is increasingly the topic of newscasts and literature. The public is demanding more information pertinent to the maintenance of health and to the ways in which the average person can act independently to do so. Health promotion is centered on ideal personal habits, lifestyles, and environmental control that decrease the risk for disease. The U.S. Public Health Service periodically identifies national health goals and most recently published a program called *Healthy People 2030*, with measurable goals to increase the general quality and years of life for all and to increase the health status of all groups to an equal level of wellness. Health promotion programs in the community are now offered by workplaces, clinics, schools, and churches, not just by hospitals as in the past.

HEALTHY PEOPLE 2030

The 5 **main goals** of *Healthy People 2030* are

- Attaining healthy, thriving lives free of preventable disease, disability, injury, and premature death
- Eliminating health disparities, achieving health equality, and increasing health literacy
- Creating environments conducive to health-promotion
- Improving health in all life stages
- Collaborating with leadership and key stakeholders in policy design that improves the health and well-being of all

Healthy People 2030 has 62 topic areas with 355 total objectives divided across five sections:

- Health Conditions
- Health Behaviors
- Populations
- Settings and Systems
- Social Determinants of Health

MAIN COMPONENTS OF HEALTH PROMOTION

Health promotion efforts are concentrated in four areas:

- Individuals must be educated to realize that their **lifestyle and choices** have a large impact on their health. They must then be motivated to choose to modify their personal risk factors and take the responsibility to do so.
- The emphasis on **good nutrition** as the biggest factor that impacts health and the length of life must be brought into general awareness. This is occurring via the media through numerous books and articles educating people about the essential nutrients needed to maintain health.
- **Stress** is a constant in a production-driven society. Individuals must learn ways to manage and decrease stress to achieve and maintain health and to decrease the effects of stress upon chronic illness, risk of infections, and trauma.
- **Physical fitness** helps cardiovascular status, relieves stress, controls weight, delays aging, promotes strength and endurance, and improves appearance and performance. Individuals must have programs that increase activity gradually to prevent injury and are designed to meet individual needs.

HEALTH SELF-MANAGEMENT

Health self-management includes health maintenance, disease prevention, and health promotion. Health maintenance is defined as strategies that help maintain and/or improve health over time. Health maintenance is dependent on three factors, which include health perception, motivation for behavioral change, and compliance to set goals. Disease prevention is an effort to limit the development or progression of lifestyle-related illness. **Disease prevention** can be categorized into primary, secondary, and tertiary prevention.

- **Primary prevention** measures are employed prior to disease onset and are used in health populations.
- **Secondary prevention** measures are used to screen, detect, and treat disease in earlier stages to prevent further progression or development of other complications.
- **Tertiary prevention** measures are used to prevent the onset of other complications or comorbid conditions.

Health promotion strategies include risk reduction strategies applied to the general population.

INFLUENCES ON DECISION TO MODIFY BEHAVIOR TO ACHIEVE AND MAINTAIN HEALTH

Many factors have an influence on people's efforts to change behavior in a way that improves and maintains their health status. These factors include age, ethnicity, gender, lifestyle, level of education, self-esteem, motivation, and self-image. The patient's support network and the availability of health promotion programs and healthcare systems also have an influence on healthcare behaviors. Some people may be prevented from accessing health promotion programs because of lack of medical insurance. Financial status and employment are important as well. The presence of addictions and diseases, the length of illness, and the severity of disabilities are all factors to be considered. The value placed on health, the threat of potential losses, and the perceived benefits of behavior modification are important motivating factors.

STRATEGIES TO ENCOURAGE SMOKING CESSATION

The **health impact associated with smoking** varies among smokers and can be affected by the number of cigarettes used daily, exposure to smoking-associated stimuli, and educational level. The presence of stress and depression, psychosocial problems, lack of coping mechanisms, low income, and long-term habitual behavior are problematic for the quitter. Nurses can promote smoking cessation by taking every opportunity to bring up the subject, educating about the dangers of smoking and benefits of quitting, and providing **resources** to help patients quit. Strategies include:

- Educating about the personal effects of smoking upon that individual
- Encouraging patients to set a quit date
- Referring to programs and smoking cessation information
- Educating about the use of nicotine replacements including nicotine gum, lozenges, inhalers, transdermal patches, and nasal sprays
- Educating about the use of medications such as Zyban®, Catapres®, and Chantix®
- Providing support via phone calls or office visits
- Discovering the reason for relapses
- Praising and rewarding any success in the quitting process

HEALTHY NUTRITION PRINCIPLES

Healthy nutrition principles include the following:

- Eating a range of different kinds of foods, and eating increased amounts fruits, vegetables, whole grains, poultry, and fish.
- Diets should consist of 55-60% **carbohydrates**, less than 30% **fat**, and the rest should be **protein** (0.8-1.0 g/kg).
- Restrict **saturated fat** to <10%. Restrict **cholesterol** to 300 mg/day.
- Utilize moderate amounts of sugar, salt, and sodium.

- Take a **multivitamin** including folic acid if the patient is female and able to have children. Get 200-800 IU/day of vitamin D in order to absorb calcium.
- **Calcium** intake should be: 1300 mg/day for women age 13-18 or those who are pregnant/nursing; 1000 mg/day for women age 19-50 years; 1500 mg/day for age 51 years and older.
- Patients who are pregnant or having chemotherapy should not try to lose weight.
- **Weight loss** may improve diabetes, joint pain, inflammation, cardiovascular disease, hypothyroidism, or renal disease.

DISEASE PREVENTION FOR THE ELDERLY

Although life spans are longer, **ongoing (chronic) diseases** are still the primary reason patients die. Elderly patients have more of an absolute chance of getting a disease, but they also react well to prevention. Keep good records of the elderly patient's history, including updating every year and following advice for patients over the age of 65 years. Evaluate nutrition, functional ability, alcoholic beverage intake (more than 2 alcoholic beverages a day constitutes abuse), smoking, illegal drugs, misuse of prescriptions, and exercise level.

- **Preventative measures** include a physical, screening assessments, and immunizations.
- Some **routine screenings** include: fasting glucose, papanicolaou smear, dipstick urinalysis, mammography, PPD, fecal occult blood/sigmoidoscopy, electrocardiogram, thyroid function, glaucoma and sight, hearing, and cholesterol.
- **Immunizations** include yearly flu shot, pneumococcal vaccine, and tetanus.

The following screens are controversial: depression for someone with no symptoms, dementia for someone with no symptoms, osteoporosis including bone densitometry for postmenopausal females (counsel females regarding hormone prophylaxis), colon and prostate cancer, and cholesterol for someone with no symptoms.

HEALTH SCREENING

YOUNG ADULT SCREENINGS

Health screening is encouraged for conditions that are very likely to occur and diseases that are likely to kill if they are not identified. The assessment should be trustworthy using proper techniques and proper follow-up.

Young adult (ages 20-39 years) screenings, according to the U.S. Preventive Services Task Force (USPSTF), should include:

- A full head-to-toe physical (every 5-6 years)
- Blood pressure screening (every 3-5 years if range is within normal: <130/85 mmHg)
- Cholesterol screening (every 5 years; more frequently when total cholesterol is higher than 200 mg/dL)
- PPD test for tuberculosis when patient has had known contact with TB or is at increased risk (health care workers, prisoners, homeless, or immunocompromised)
- Dental check-up (annually)
- Thyroid palpation (every 3 years)
- Depression screening (at every visit)
- Men perform self-testicular exam every month
- Women conduct a self-breast exam every month; should receive a clinical breast exam every 3 years

- Pap smear and pelvic assessments every 3-years (or up to 5 years in conjunction with HPV testing)
- Screening for gonorrhea and chlamydia for all sexually active individuals
- Health education and promotion (every time patient is seen)
- Influenza vaccination (annually)
- Td immunization every 10 years

Adult Screenings

Adults (age 40 and older) screenings, according to the USPSTF, should maintain the same schedule as young adults (unless indicated below) in addition to the following:

- A full head-to-toe physical (annually)
- Blood pressure screening (annually)
- ECG (over 40, annually; only when there are cardiac risks)
- Clinical breast exam (annually in women over 40)
- Mammogram (biennially in women over 50)
- General colorectal cancer screening for risks (annually), and colorectal cancer screening via colonoscopy (every 10 years for those over 50 until age 75)
- Prostate-specific antigen screening (men over 50 with average risk, or younger if higher risk; upon the patient's informed request only)

NP Primary Care Practice Test

1. If the Adult NP wanted to incorporate the transtheoretical model into an educational plan, what would be the first step?
   a. Preparation.
   b. Precontemplation.
   c. Contemplation.
   d. Action.

2. A 70-year-old female with Alzheimer's and a history of falls is admitted to the unit with pneumonitis after a seven-hour wait in the emergency department. The patient is agitated, restless, and repeatedly says "I'm hungry." The nurse's first priority should be to:
   a. assess diet needs and order food.
   b. institute a fall-prevention program.
   c. review all medications.
   d. assess cognitive abilities.

3. Which of the following techniques should be used when interviewing an elderly woman?
   a. Speak quickly to get through a focused assessment before the woman tires.
   b. Speak in a quiet and calming tone so that the woman does not become agitated.
   c. Speak loudly and clearly so that the woman can hear you.
   d. Perform the interview with the company primary caregiver to have help clarifying issues if necessary.

4. A 77-year-old male patient has increasing dementia with short-term memory loss and symptoms that fluctuate frequently. The patient experiences visual hallucinations and exhibits muscle rigidity and tremors. These symptoms are characteristic of which type of non-Alzheimer's dementia?
   a. Dementia with Lewy bodies.
   b. Frontotemporal dementia.
   c. Normal pressure hydrocephalus.
   d. Parkinson's dementia.

5. According to Becker, which of the following factors plays a large role in influencing a patient's health?
   a. Education.
   b. Income.
   c. Family support.
   d. Language spoken.

6. A woman complains of a history of nausea and burning, stabbing epigastric pain which is relieved for short periods by antacids or intake of food. The patient denies NSAID use but is a heavy smoker. A urea breath test is positive. Which of the following treatment protocols is most common?
   a. Histamine-2 blocker plus bismuth plus tetracycline.
   b. Proton pump inhibitor only.
   c. Proton pump inhibitor plus tetracycline.
   d. Proton pump inhibitor plus clarithromycin and amoxicillin/metronidazole.

7. Which of the following is the best documentation of the behavior of a difficult patient?
    a. "Patient is belligerent and uncooperative."
    b. "Patient is spitting at nurses, throwing magazines, and refusing to get out of bed for therapy."
    c. "Patient appears to dislike nurses and other care providers."
    d. "Patient believes staff members are going to hurt her."

8. According to the *Dietary Guidelines for Americans, 2010*, the sodium restriction for those who are 51 years and older, African American, or with existing cardiovascular disease, renal disease, or diabetes is:
    a. <2300 mg/day.
    b. 1500 mg/day.
    c. <300 mg/day.
    d. <1000 mg/day.

9. Who determines an APRN's right to write prescriptions?
    a. Standards of Practice.
    b. The American Nursing Association.
    c. The state where the APRN is practicing.
    d. The Drug Enforcement Agency.

10. A patient's laboratory tests show that the TSH is 14 mU/mL, free T4 is 3.5 µg/dL and free T3 is 100 ng/dL. These findings indicate:
    a. normal values.
    b. hypothyroidism.
    c. hyperthyroidism.
    d. Hashimoto's thyroiditis.

11. What type of research involves analyzing how well a medical treatment is progressing?
    a. Causation.
    b. Meta-analysis.
    c. Therapeutic.
    d. Systemic review.

12. An incidence of which of the following conditions requires mandatory reporting to the CDC?
    a. Influenza.
    b. Lyme disease.
    c. Hepatitis E.
    d. Methicillin-resistant Staphylococcus aureus infection.

13. When obtaining consent for a patient participating in a research study, what is the most important step for the nurse to make sure was completed?
    a. Ensure safety of the treatment.
    b. Consent was obtained, including a statement guaranteeing a patient's privacy and confidentiality.
    c. Double-blind conditions are maintained.
    d. That the patient is aware of which treatment he is receiving.

14. In evidence-based research, what do persistent erratic findings in tracking and trending suggest?
   a. Changes in patient population requiring changes in processes of care.
   b. Errors in statistical analysis of processes of care.
   c. Normal day-to-day variations in processes of care.
   d. Processes of care are not consistent or are inadequate.

15. Total quality management (TQM) is different from quality assurance (QA) because:
   a. QA is best accomplished through peer review and TQM should be based on observations from the managing supervisor.
   b. TQM is best accomplished through peer review and QA should be based on observations from the managing supervisor.
   c. QA occurs continuously; TQM happens only periodically.
   d. TQM occurs continuously; QA happens only periodically.

16. A patient with severe type 1 diabetes mellitus refuses all treatment because of religious convictions. Which of the following is the most appropriate action?
   a. Provide the patient with facts about the disease, treatments, and prognosis.
   b. Ask family members to intervene.
   c. Remind the patient that he will die without treatment.
   d. Refer the patient to a psychologist.

17. Which of the following groups MUST be covered under Medicaid?
   a. Persons who are eligible for Aid to Families with Dependent Children.
   b. Persons older than 40 years with a disability.
   c. Persons older than 65 years without a disability.
   d. Children born after 1990 living in families below the poverty line.

18. A 64-year-old female presents with bilateral ptosis and diplopia, slurred speech, increasing generalized weakness (which decreases with rest), and dysphagia. Based on these findings, the nurse practitioner suspects:
   a. stroke.
   b. myasthenia gravis.
   c. multiple sclerosis.
   d. Parkinson's disease.

19. Which of the following statements is CORRECT about Medicaid?
   a. Everyone who falls below the federal poverty line is eligible to receive Medicaid.
   b. The state is allowed to require that recipients pay a small copayment.
   c. Recipients of Medicaid are not supposed to pay anything towards their medical care.
   d. Though it is both a federal and state plan, only the state government is responsible for supervision of the program.

20. When the nurse practitioner enters the room of a patient whose death is imminent, the daughter states, "I can't stay in the room when Dad dies! I can't stand the thought!" Which of the following is the best response?
    a. "You will regret it if you don't."
    b. "Your father would want you with him."
    c. "I'll stay with him, and you can come and go as you feel comfortable."
    d. "Is there someone else who can stay with him?"

21. Negligence is:
    a. Not acting in a way that a reasonable and prudent nurse would, resulting in harm to the patient.
    b. Acting in a way that is against the law, resulting in harm to the patient.
    c. not taking the appropriate preventative measures that another nurse would, to the detriment of the patient.
    d. not giving appropriate medical care to a patient.

22. Which of the following communication approaches is most effective to facilitate communication with a patient who has global aphasia?
    a. Speak slowly and clearly, facing the patient.
    b. Use letter boards.
    c. Ask yes/no questions.
    d. Use pictures, diagrams, and gestures.

23. A thin young adult comes into the emergency room with a sudden onset of right-sided chest pain and shortness of breath following a run. What do you suspect?
    a. Myocardial infarction.
    b. Aortic dissection.
    c. Asthma flare.
    d. Spontaneous pneumothorax.

24. A staff nurse reports that she has provided a patient with written instructions about wound care, but the patient states repeatedly that she hasn't read the material. The nurse practitioner should advise the staff nurse to:
    a. provide alternative materials, such as videos.
    b. do a vision and literacy assessment.
    c. advise the patient again that she needs to read the material.
    d. ask the patient why she is not cooperating.

25. A young woman presents in the emergency room with sudden shortness of breath, coughing, and slight chest pain. She is on the birth control pill and just returned home from a car trip several hours away. What tests should you order?
    a. ABG, ECG, chest x-ray, and echocardiogram.
    b. CBC, pulmonary function test, stress test.
    c. ECG, cardiac enzymes, stress test.
    d. Sputum culture, CBC, pulmonary function test.

26. When determining the burden of proof for acts of negligence, how would risk management classify willfully providing inadequate care while disregarding the safety and security of another?
    a. Negligent conduct.
    b. Gross negligence.
    c. Contributory negligence.
    d. Comparative negligence.

27. In a patient with severe dyslipidemia, what physical changes might you expect to see?
    a. Velvety skin behind the neck.
    b. Cyanotic fingernails.
    c. Opaque corneas and xanthomas.
    d. Bulging eyes.

28. When the nurse practitioner is conducting medication reconciliation, the patient's list of current medications includes the following: Lasix®, metolazone, aminophylline, and doxapram. The nurse believes this list probably indicates:
    a. polypharmacy.
    b. inaccurate reporting.
    c. accurate reporting.
    d. poor medical management.

29. Brudzinski sign and Kernig sign are both indications of:
    a. carpal tunnel syndrome.
    b. DVT.
    c. Cushing syndrome.
    d. meningitis.

30. Which of the following sensory changes associated with aging has the most impact on older adults?
    a. Hearing deficit.
    b. Vision deficit.
    c. Decreased taste and smell.
    d. Decreased sense of touch (vibration, temperature, pain).

31. A thyroid panel comes back with the following results: elevated TSH, low free T4, and low free T3. What is the diagnosis?
    a. Hyperthyroidism.
    b. Subclinical hypothyroidism.
    c. Primary hypothyroidism.
    d. Subclinical hyperthyroidism.

32. With the Timed Up and Go (TUG) test to assess ambulation and mobility, which completion time indicates increased risk for falls?
    a. 10 seconds.
    b. 8 seconds.
    c. 14 seconds.
    d. 5 seconds.

33. At what age should men begin having yearly PSA tests?
    a. When a man expresses a desire for the screening and understands the risks and benefits.
    b. Starting at age 40.
    c. Starting at age 50.
    d. Starting at age 60.

34. When prescribing an oral anti-diabetic agent for an older patient, the patient's initial dose should be:
    a. the same as the usual dose for a younger adult.
    b. 25% of the usual dose.
    c. 50% of the usual dose.
    d. 75% of the usual dose.

35. Which of the following is not a necessary test for a 40-year-old woman at her yearly checkup?
    a. Mammogram.
    b. Clinical breast exam.
    c. Glaucoma screening.
    d. Colon cancer screening.

36. When a patient is following DASH (dietary approaches to stop hypertension), total fat should comprise what percentage of the diet?
    a. 6%.
    b. 55%.
    c. 18%.
    d. 27%.

37. What is the antibiotic of choice in a patient with syphilis, who reports an allergy to penicillin?
    a. Doxycycline 100 mg PO BID x 14 days.
    b. Ofloxacin 400 mg PO BID x 14 days.
    c. Ceftriaxone 250 mg IM x 1 dose.
    d. Metronidazole 500 mg PO BID x 14 days.

38. A patient is being treated for malnutrition with increased caloric and protein intake. Which of the following laboratory tests is best for assessing short-term changes in nutritional status?
    a. Total protein.
    b. Albumin.
    c. Prealbumin.
    d. Transferrin.

39. After performing a Papanicolaou test (Pap smear) on a patient, the results indicate ASCUS, atypical squamous cells of undetermined significance. What is the recommended course of action?
    a. Nothing, this is an insignificant result.
    b. Repeat the pap in 4 to 6 months.
    c. Immediate colposcopy and biopsy.
    d. Referral to an oncologist.

40. Which of the following regulatory guidelines contains the Nursing Home Reform Amendments, which establish guidelines for long-term care facilities?
    a. Omnibus Budget Reconciliation Act (OBRA).
    b. Older Americans Act (OAA).
    c. Americans with Disabilities Act (ADA).
    d. Health Insurance Portability and Accountability Act (HIPAA).

41. Which drug that is used for the treatment of coronary artery disease should be avoided in patients with asthma?
    a. Spironolactone.
    b. Losartan.
    c. Propranolol.
    d. Captopril.

42. A 76-year-old male is recovering from surgery but exhibits sudden onset of confusion with fluctuating inattention, disorganized thinking, and altered level of consciousness. Which of the following assessment tools is most indicated?
    a. Mini-mental state exam (MMSE).
    b. Mini-Cog.
    c. Confusion assessment method (CAM).
    d. Geriatric depression scale (GDS).

43. Losartan works by:
    a. preventing conversion of angiotensin I to angiotensin II.
    b. blocking beta receptors in the heart to slow the heart rate.
    c. blocking alpha receptors in the heart to lessen contractility of the heart.
    d. removing fluid from the circulatory system through the urine.

44. When counseling a patient about the need for a herpes zoster immunization, which of the following should the nurse practitioner tell the patient?
    a. The vaccine prevents about 50% of cases and decreases pain and severity of those who develop disease.
    b. The immunization should be routinely administered to those who are immunocompromised.
    c. There are no adverse effects associated with the immunization.
    d. The immunization is recommended for those 50 years and older.

45. Which antibiotic should be avoided in patients taking theophylline?
    a. Doxycycline.
    b. Erythromycin.
    c. Vancomycin.
    d. Penicillin.

46. A 60-year-old male has had yearly negative fecal occult blood tests. The nurse practitioner should advise him to have a colonoscopy:
    a. every year.
    b. every 5 years.
    c. every 10 years.
    d. every 2 years until age 70.

47. In patients taking valproic acid for seizure disorder, serum levels should be maintained at:
   a. 50 to 100 mcg/mL.
   b. 20 to 80 mcg/mL.
   c. 10 to 20 mcg/mL.
   d. 4 to 12 mcg/mL.

48. A woman has had stable angina for four years, with pain resolving within three to four minutes with rest and sublingual nitroglycerin, but the patient reports a sudden change: pain is more intense, lasts longer, occurs at rest, and is unrelieved by one nitroglycerin. The nurse practitioner should:
   a. prescribe a long-acting vasodilator.
   b. order ECG and cardiac enzyme studies to evaluate condition.
   c. advise the patient to increase frequency of nitroglycerin administration.
   d. immediately refer the patient for emergent cardiac care.

49. Which of the following is NOT an example of a HAART regimen of HIV medications?
   a. Efavirenz along with two nucleoside reverse transcriptase inhibitors (NRTIs).
   b. Indinavir along with two NRTIs.
   c. Nelfinavir along with two NRTIs.
   d. Two NRTIs.

50. An alert but frail and forgetful 80-year-old female has lost weight and had two recent falls when she was left alone while her daughter, with whom she lives, went to work (three days a week from 9 AM to 4 PM). The best referral is:
   a. Meals on Wheels.
   b. long-term care facility.
   c. adult protective services.
   d. adult day care.

Answer Key and Explanations

1. B: The transtheoretical model of health education was developed by Prochaska and Velicer in 1997. The steps, in order, are precontemplation, contemplation, preparation, action, and, finally, maintenance of the behavior.

2. A: The first priority should be to attend to the patient's comfort needs by assessing diet needs, including food allergies, and ordering food. Because the patient has a history of falls, the nurse practitioner should institute a program of fall prevention, assessing the best methods to prevent injury to the patient. The nurse should then review all medications to ensure that no ongoing medical needs are overlooked, as patients may not provide full information in the emergency department. Cognitive abilities are best assessed when the patient is comfortable and rested.

3. C: Speaking quickly or quietly may make it difficult for the woman to hear you. If possible, the interview should be performed outside of the presence of the primary caregiver so you can properly screen for elder abuse. If this is not possible, at least perform that part of the screening while the patient is alone. When interviewing an elderly woman, you should speak in a clear voice at an adequate volume, while facing the patient. Watch for signs that she is tiring or becoming stressed and adjust your technique accordingly, or take a break if necessary.

4. A: These symptoms are characteristic of dementia with Lewy bodies. Cognitive and physical decline is similar to Alzheimer's, but symptoms may fluctuate frequently. This form of dementia may include visual hallucinations, muscle rigidity, and tremors. Frontotemporal dementia may cause marked changes in personality and behavior and is characterized by difficulty using and understanding language. Normal pressure hydrocephalus is characterized by ataxia, memory loss, and urinary incontinence. Parkinson's dementia may involve impaired decision making and difficulty concentrating, learning new material, understanding complex language, and sequencing as well as inflexibility and short- or long-term memory loss.

5. B: According to Becker, health depends on a patient's age, gender, race, ethnicity, and salary or income. Education, family support, and spoken language are not included in his list of factors that impact a person's health.

6. D: These symptoms are consistent with a duodenal ulcer, and the positive urea breath test indicates a *Helicobacter pylori* infection, which is usually treated with a proton pump inhibitor plus clarithromycin and amoxicillin/metronidazole. About 90% of duodenal ulcers are associated with *H. pylori* infection. *H. pylori* weakens the mucosa and results in hypersecretion of gastric acid. Eating may increase pain with gastric ulcers but usually relieves pain with duodenal ulcers. Smoking increases the risk of peptic ulcer disease, and use of NSAIDs increases risk of serious complications, such as bleeding or perforation.

7. B: "Patient is spitting at nurses, throwing magazines, and refusing to get out of bed for therapy" describes the patient's behavior without placing a value judgment ("belligerent and uncooperative"), which might indicate bias against the patient. The nurse should avoid interpreting behavior ("appears to dislike") or characterizing what's in a patient's mind ("Patient believes"). Patients, especially older adults or those who are confused, may behave in a difficult manner if they are afraid, in pain, or overwhelmed, so the nurse should attempt to find the reason for the behavior.

8. B: 1500 mg/day.

Sodium: <2300 mg/day and 1500 mg/day for those ≥51 years or African American or with existing cardiovascular or renal disease or diabetes.
Saturated fat: <10% of calories.
Dietary cholesterol: <300 mg/day.

Alcohol: ≤1 drink daily for women and ≤2 for men.

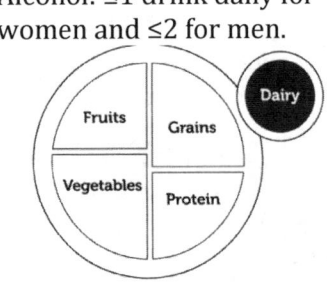

Use lower fat milk products.
Eat a variety of high protein foods, including seafood, beans, and nuts.
Replace solid fats with oils.
Limit trans fatty acids, solid fats, sugar, and refined grains.

9. C: The ability to write prescriptions is dictated by the scope of practice, which is set by the state in which the nurse is practicing.

10. B: These laboratory findings indicate hypothyroidism, which is characterized by increased TSH, decreased free T4, and normal free T3. Normal values for an older adult:

- TSH: 0.32–5.0 mU/mL.
- Free T4: 4.5–12 µg/dL
- Free T3: 75–200 ng/dL.

Hyperthyroidism is characterized by decreased TSH (<0.30), increased free T4 and increased T3. Additional tests may be indicated for those with comorbidities and multiple medications. Thyroid autoantibody tests are used to help diagnose Hashimoto's thyroiditis.

11. C: This is an example of a therapeutic research study; it analyzes how a medical treatment is progressing. These studies are often random and double-blind, and utilize a placebo. Causation studies check to see if a chemical or drug is harmful or connected to a particular health problem. Both systemic reviews and meta-analysis studies look at other research to summarize other studies, though each in a different manner.

12. B: Lyme disease requires mandatory reporting while reporting of the other diseases is voluntary. The CDC maintains a reportable disease list, which is upgraded and revised as necessary and reissued July 1 of each year. Each state also maintains a reportable disease list, which may or may not be identical with that of the CDC, so the nurse must be familiar with all reportable disease requirements. Much data at the state and local level is confidential name-based information, but data collected at the CDC is without names or personal identifying information. Some states require reporting of hospital-acquired infections.

13. B: When obtaining consent from a patient who is participating in a research study, the statement guaranteeing patient privacy and confidentiality must be in the consent form. By law, if not included in the statement, the consent is not valid.

14. D: While trends will show some normal variation, if the trend becomes erratic and measures are inconsistent, this suggests that the processes of care are not consistent or are inadequate. Tracking and trending is central to developing research-supported evidence-based practice and is part of continuous quality improvement. Once processes and outcomes measurements are selected, then at least one measure should be tracked for a number of periods of time, usually in increments of four weeks or quarterly. This tracking can be used to present graphical representation of results that will show trends.

15. D: Both QA and TQM can be accomplished by either a peer review process or by observations made by the managing supervisor. The difference between QA and TQM is that QA only occurs periodically, while TQM is an ongoing process.

16. A: Patients have a right to refuse treatment for religious or other personal reasons, so the most appropriate action is to simply provide the patient with factual information about the disease, treatments, and prognosis in a neutral manner, without trying to coerce or frighten the patient. In some cases, patients may change their minds when presented with information, but the nurse should remain supportive regardless of the patient's decision. Asking the family to intervene is not appropriate and refusal of treatment alone does not suggest the need for referral to a psychologist.

17. A: At a minimum, persons must be living under the poverty line to qualify for Medicaid. However, not everyone who satisfies that requirement will receive aid. Persons who are eligible for Aid to Families with Dependent Children, patients older than 65 years with a disability, and children born after 1983 living in families below the poverty line must receive assistance under federal guidelines. People older than 65 years qualify for Medicare, not Medicaid.

18. B: Myasthenia gravis (MG) is an autoimmune disorder of the neuromuscular system in which acetylcholine receptors are damaged at neural synapses, preventing transmission of impulses to contract muscles. The thymus gland develops abnormalities and sometimes thymoma. Symptoms of MG include muscle weakness, which decreases with rest. Eye muscles are often affected first, resulting in ptosis and visual disturbances such as diplopia. General weakness in extremities, neck, and face as well as dysphagia and slurred speech occur. Acute respiratory failure can occur as part of myasthenic crisis before diagnosis or in relation to fever, infection, or drug therapy.

19. B: Medicaid is not always completely free for those who receive aid. Though they cannot bill recipients for medical care, the state is allowed by the federal government to charge a small co-pay. Not everyone who lives below the federal poverty guidelines will qualify for Medicaid. Medicaid is overseen by both the state and federal governments.

20. C: The nurse practitioner should remain supportive and nonjudgmental. "I'll stay with him, and you can come and go as you feel comfortable" supports the daughter's stated desire while still leaving open the opportunity for her to spend time with her father during the death vigil. People react in very different ways to death, and many people have never seen a deceased person and may be very frightened. While many people find comfort in being with a dying friend or family member, this should never be imposed on anyone.

21. A: The definition of negligence is when a medical professional acts in a way that a reasonable person of the same education and skill level would not, and this action results in patient harm. Disloyalty, acting in an illegal manner, or not acting at all to prevent a patient from being harmed is called malpractice.

22. D: Aphasia is the loss of ability to use and/or understand written and spoken language because of damage to the speech center of the brain caused by brain tumors, brain injury, and stroke. Global aphasia is characterized by difficulty understanding and producing language in speaking, reading, and writing although patients may understand gestures. The nurse can use pictures, diagrams, and gestures to convey meaning. Picture charts are also useful. The speech pathologist should assess patients with aphasia and provide guidance in communicating with them.

23. D: Young, thin males are particularly prone to spontaneous pneumothorax, especially following exercise. Shortness of breath would not be present in patients having an aortic dissection, and chest pain would be on the left side if they were having an MI. Asthma generally does not cause chest pain.

24. B: The nurse practitioner should do a vision and literacy assessment to ensure the patient is able to read, because the patient may be reluctant to admit the inability to read the material. Written materials for older adults should be age appropriate, clearly written with a large font size, and illustrated. Videos are a useful adjunct to teaching as they reduce the time needed for one-on-one instruction (increasing cost effectiveness). Videos are much more effective than written materials for those with low literacy or poor English skills. The nurse should always be available to answer questions and discuss the material after the patients/families finish viewing.

25. A: Given her history, you should immediately suspect that she has a pulmonary embolus, or a blood clot that passed into the lung tissue. You should order an ABG to assess oxygenation, and an ECG and chest x-ray to rule out other causative conditions.

26. B: Gross negligence. Negligence indicates that *proper care* has not been provided, based on established standards. *Reasonable care* uses rationale for decision-making in relation to providing care. Types of negligence:

- Negligent conduct indicates that an individual failed to provide reasonable care or to protect/assist another, based on standards and expertise.
- Gross negligence is willfully providing inadequate care while disregarding the safety and security of another.
- Contributory negligence involves the injured party contributing to his or her own harm.
- Comparative negligence attempts to determine what percentage amount of negligence is attributed to each individual involved.

27. C: The excess fatty material in the blood could manifest as opaque corneas and xanthomas, small fatty deposits most commonly found on the eyelid. Velvety skin behind the neck indicates insulin resistance or early diabetes. Cyanotic fingernails are a sign of poor oxygenation, and bulging eyes could be a sign of thyroid disease.

28. A: Since Lasix® and metolazone are both diuretics and aminophylline and doxapram are both methylxanthines, this list probably indicates polypharmacy. Older adults are especially at risk for polypharmacy—taking too many drugs—because of taking the same drug under generic and brand names, taking drugs for one condition but contraindicated for another, and taking drugs that are not compatible. Reasons for polypharmacy include multiple prescriptions from different doctors; forgetfulness; confusion; failure to report current medications; the use of supplemental, over-the-counter, and herbal preparations in addition to prescribed medications; and failure of healthcare providers to adequately educate the patient.

29. D: Brudzinski sign occurs when there is severe neck stiffness. When the neck is flexed, the hips and knees also flex to compensate for the decreased movement; this is considered to be a positive result. A positive Kernig sign results when there is stiffness and discomfort in the hamstrings, making the patient unable to straighten their legs when the hip is flexed to 90 degrees. Both signs indicate meningitis.

30. B: Older adults are most impacted by deteriorating vision (presbyopia, cataracts), which prevents them from reading and navigating safely. Most people older than 60 require glasses.

People may be less sensitive to color differences (particularly blues and greens), and night vision decreases. Hearing impairment (impacted cerumen, presbycusis) may require periodic cleaning of the ears or hearing aids. Taste and smell usually remain fairly intact although smell of airborne chemicals may be less acute, and taste buds begin to atrophy around age 60, affecting the ability to taste sweet and salt especially. The sense of touch is usually somewhat reduced in older adults.

31. C: When the TSH is elevated, it is an indication that the thyroid is in a sluggish (i.e., hypothyroid) state and needs higher amounts of TSH to stimulate production of the thyroid hormones. In primary hypothyroidism, both levels of free T4 and free T3 are low. In cases of subclinical hypothyroidism, free T3 and free T4 are not affected, and their levels remain within the normal range.

32. C: Timed Up and Go (TUG): Patient stands from chair with armrests, walks 3 meters, and turns and sits back down. Those requiring ≥14 seconds are at risk for falls (normal: 7–10 seconds). During assessment, the patient should be carefully observed for gait abnormalities, including unsteadiness, uneven weight distribution, abnormal position of limbs, and type of gait. Gait assessment also includes:

- Gait speed in 5 meters with slow gait (<0.6 m/second) predictive of functional limitations.
- Performance oriented mobility assessment (POMA) tests mobility and gait under different conditions.

33. A: Recommendations regarding PSA screening have recently changed. The American Academy of Family Physicians (AAFP) now recommends against routine PSA screening. This change is due to evidence that, while screening for PSA can decrease the mortality rate of prostate cancer for a small population of men, there are also long-term risk associated, including erectile dysfunction and urinary incontinence. These risks may outweigh the benefits of the screening, depending on the patient. The AAFP recommends, for men ages 55-69 with a family history or individual risk factors for prostate cancer and request screening, that information be provided regarding the benefits and risks to allow the patient to make an informed decision on the screening. The AAFP recommends against PSA screening in men ages 70 due to the likelihood that men over 70 are more likely to die due to other health issues.

34. C: 50%. Problems associated with older adults and different types of drugs:

Anti-diabetics	Oral anti-diabetic agents should be started at 50% of the usual dose because of the danger of hypoglycemia. First generation drugs should be avoided. Glucotrol® has fewer side effects than Diabeta®.
Antidepressants	Antidepressants are associated with excess sedation, so typical doses are only 16–33% of a younger adult's dose. SSRIs are safest, but Prozac® should be avoided because it may cause anorexia, anxiety, and insomnia.
Anticoagulants	Anticoagulants may cause severe bleeding in those over 65. Warfarin should be used with care and at a lower dose if total protein or albumin concentration is low.

35. D: Colon cancer screenings are not necessary, unless the patient has a strong family history or multiple risk factors, or is symptomatic, until the age of 50. Yearly mammograms and glaucoma screenings should begin at age 40, and a physician should be performing the clinical breast exam every year beginning with a woman's first gynecological appointment.

36. D: DASH nutrient goals (based on a 2100 calorie diet) include:

Total fat 27%, saturated fat 6%, protein 18%, carbohydrates 55%, cholesterol 150 mg, Na 1500–2300 mg, K 4700 mg, Ca 1250 mg, Mg 500 mg, fiber 3 g.

Food group	Daily servings
Grains (whole grains preferred)	6–8
Vegetables and fruits	4–5 each
Fat-free or low-fat milk/milk products	2–3
Lean meat, poultry, fish	≤6 (serving = 1 ounce)
Nuts, seeds, legumes	4–5 per week
Fats and oils	2–3
Sweets and added sugars	≤5 per week

37. A: Except for neurosyphilis, the primary treatment should be penicillin G 2.4 million units IM for one dose. In patients who are allergic to penicillin, the treatment of choice is doxycycline 100 mg PO twice a day for 14 days OR tetracycline 500 mg PO four times a day for 14 days. Pregnant patients are an exception; they should still be given penicillin after undergoing desensitization.

38. C: Prealbumin (transthyretin) is most commonly monitored for acute changes in nutritional status because it has a half-life of only 2–3 days.

- Normal values: 16–40 mg/dL
- Mild deficiency: 10–15 mg/dL
- Moderate deficiency: 5–9 mg/dL
- Severe deficiency: <5 mg/dL

Total protein can be influenced by many factors, including stress and infection. Albumin is the most common screening to determine protein levels. Albumin has a half-life of 18–20 days, so it is sensitive to long-term protein deficiencies. Transferrin is not always a reliable measurement of nutritional status because levels are affected by many factors.

39. B: ASCUS (atypical squamous cells of undetermined significance) means that the cells are not the typical squamocolumnar cervical cells or endocervical glandular cells that you would expect to see in a Pap smear. It does not, however, mean that the cells are dysplastic. The test should be repeated in 4 to 6 months to see if there are any changes.

40. A: Omnibus Budget Reconciliation Act (OBRA): Contains the Nursing Home Reform Amendments (NHRA), which establish guidelines for nursing facilities (such as long-term care facilities). Older Americans Act (OAA): Provides improved access to services for older adults and Native Americans, including community services (meals, transportation, home health care, adult day care, legal assistance, and home repair). Americans with Disabilities Act (ADA): Civil rights legislation that provides the disabled, including those with mental impairment, access to employment and the community. Health Insurance Portability and Accountability Act (HIPAA): Addresses the rights of the individual related to privacy of health information.

41. C: Propranolol is a beta-blocker and reduces myocardial demand for oxygen. It also can cause bronchospasm and should be avoided in patients who have any form of bronchospastic disease, such as asthma.

42. C: CAM: Assesses development of delirium. Factors indicative of delirium include:

- Onset: Acute change in mental status.
- Attention: Inattentive, stable, or fluctuating.
- Thinking: Disorganized, rambling conversation, switching topics, illogical.
- Level of consciousness: Altered, ranging from alert to coma.
- Orientation: Disoriented (person, place, time).
- Memory: Impaired.
- Perceptual disturbances: Hallucinations, illusions.
- Psychomotor abnormalities: Agitation (tapping, picking, moving) or retardation (staring, not moving).
- Sleep-wake cycle: Awake at night and sleepy in the daytime.

MMSE and Mini-Cog are used to assess evidence of dementia or short-term memory loss, often associated with Alzheimer's disease. GDS is a self-assessment tool to identify older adults with depression.

43. A: Losartan is an angiotensin receptor blocker (ARB) and works by preventing the conversion of angiotensin I to angiotensin II, to lower blood pressure. In addition, it is an effective vasodilator. Beta-blockers and alpha-blockers block beta and alpha receptors, respectively. Diuretics remove excess fluid from the circulatory system through the urine.

44. A: The herpes zoster vaccine prevents about 50% of herpes zoster cases and decreases the pain and severity for those who still develop the disease. It is contraindicated in those with an allergy to gelatin or neomycin and those who are immunocompromised because of HIV/AIDS, chemotherapy, radiation, steroid use, history of leukemia or lymphoma, and active TB. Adverse reactions are rare but include allergic response, local inflammation, and headache. The herpes zoster vaccine is recommended for those 60 years and older.

45. B: Erythromycin lessens theophylline's effectiveness and should not be prescribed in a patient who is taking theophylline. Consider an alternate antibiotic.

46. C: Every 10 years. Screening should begin at age 50 for those with average risk and age 40 with increased risk. Screening tests:

- Colonoscopy—every 10 years or as follow-up for abnormalities in other screening; allows for removal of polyps, small cancerous lesions, and biopsies, and provides surveillance of inflammatory bowel disease.
- Fecal occult blood—yearly; checks for blood in stool.
- Flexible sigmoidoscopy—every 5 years; checks for polyps or signs of cancer in rectum and lower third of colon.
- Double contrast barium enema—every 5 years; x-ray with contrast to visualize intestinal abnormalities.

47. A: The therapeutic serum levels for valproic acid is between 50 and 100 mcg/mL. Clonazepam therapeutic serum levels are between 20 and 80 ng/mL. Carbamazepine should be maintained at serum levels of 4 to 12 mcg/mL, and phenytoin should be maintained at serum levels of 10 to 20 mcg/mL.

48. D: The nurse practitioner should refer the patient for emergent cardiac care. Unstable angina (AKA preinfarction or crescendo angina) is a progression of coronary artery disease and occurs when there is a change in the pattern of stable angina. The pain may increase, may not respond to a single nitroglycerin, and may persist for >5 minutes. Usually pain is more frequent, lasts longer, and may occur at rest. Unstable angina may indicate rupture of an atherosclerotic plaque and the beginning of thrombus formation, so it should always be treated as a medical emergency as it may indicate a myocardial infarction.

49. D: HAART drug regimens for HIV involve 3 different HIV drugs, which tend to be more effective than a single drug regimen. Choice D, only 2 NRTIs, is not a HAART regimen. In addition to the drug protocols listed in the question (choices A through C), ritonavir and indinavir along with 2 NRTIs, ritonavir and lopinavir along with 2 NRTIs, and ritonavir and saquinavir along with 2 NRTIs are all other examples of HAART drug protocols.

50. D: The best referral is to an adult day care program because the patient can be in a safe environment with meals provided while the daughter is at work. Meals on Wheels provides for meals only, but this patient's age, condition, and frailty put her at risk, so she should not be left unattended. She does not require full-time care, such as provided by a long-term care facility, since she is home with her daughter most of the time. Adult protective services are indicated only if there is evidence of abuse or neglect.

How to Overcome Test Anxiety

Just the thought of taking a test is enough to make most people a little nervous. A test is an important event that can have a long-term impact on your future, so it's important to take it seriously and it's natural to feel anxious about performing well. But just because anxiety is normal, that doesn't mean that it's helpful in test taking, or that you should simply accept it as part of your life. Anxiety can have a variety of effects. These effects can be mild, like making you feel slightly nervous, or severe, like blocking your ability to focus or remember even a simple detail.

If you experience test anxiety—whether severe or mild—it's important to know how to beat it. To discover this, first you need to understand what causes test anxiety.

Causes of Test Anxiety

While we often think of anxiety as an uncontrollable emotional state, it can actually be caused by simple, practical things. One of the most common causes of test anxiety is that a person does not feel adequately prepared for their test. This feeling can be the result of many different issues such as poor study habits or lack of organization, but the most common culprit is time management. Starting to study too late, failing to organize your study time to cover all of the material, or being distracted while you study will mean that you're not well prepared for the test. This may lead to cramming the night before, which will cause you to be physically and mentally exhausted for the test. Poor time management also contributes to feelings of stress, fear, and hopelessness as you realize you are not well prepared but don't know what to do about it.

Other times, test anxiety is not related to your preparation for the test but comes from unresolved fear. This may be a past failure on a test, or poor performance on tests in general. It may come from comparing yourself to others who seem to be performing better or from the stress of living up to expectations. Anxiety may be driven by fears of the future—how failure on this test would affect your educational and career goals. These fears are often completely irrational, but they can still negatively impact your test performance.

> **Review Video: 3 Reasons You Have Test Anxiety**
> Visit mometrix.com/academy and enter code: 428468

Elements of Test Anxiety

As mentioned earlier, test anxiety is considered to be an emotional state, but it has physical and mental components as well. Sometimes you may not even realize that you are suffering from test anxiety until you notice the physical symptoms. These can include trembling hands, rapid heartbeat, sweating, nausea, and tense muscles. Extreme anxiety may lead to fainting or vomiting. Obviously, any of these symptoms can have a negative impact on testing. It is important to recognize them as soon as they begin to occur so that you can address the problem before it damages your performance.

> **Review Video: 3 Ways to Tell You Have Test Anxiety**
> Visit mometrix.com/academy and enter code: 927847

The mental components of test anxiety include trouble focusing and inability to remember learned information. During a test, your mind is on high alert, which can help you recall information and stay focused for an extended period of time. However, anxiety interferes with your mind's natural processes, causing you to blank out, even on the questions you know well. The strain of testing during anxiety makes it difficult to stay focused, especially on a test that may take several hours. Extreme anxiety can take a huge mental toll, making it difficult not only to recall test information but even to understand the test questions or pull your thoughts together.

> **Review Video: How Test Anxiety Affects Memory**
> Visit mometrix.com/academy and enter code: 609003

Effects of Test Anxiety

Test anxiety is like a disease—if left untreated, it will get progressively worse. Anxiety leads to poor performance, and this reinforces the feelings of fear and failure, which in turn lead to poor performances on subsequent tests. It can grow from a mild nervousness to a crippling condition. If allowed to progress, test anxiety can have a big impact on your schooling, and consequently on your future.

Test anxiety can spread to other parts of your life. Anxiety on tests can become anxiety in any stressful situation, and blanking on a test can turn into panicking in a job situation. But fortunately, you don't have to let anxiety rule your testing and determine your grades. There are a number of relatively simple steps you can take to move past anxiety and function normally on a test and in the rest of life.

> **Review Video: How Test Anxiety Impacts Your Grades**
> Visit mometrix.com/academy and enter code: 939819

Physical Steps for Beating Test Anxiety

While test anxiety is a serious problem, the good news is that it can be overcome. It doesn't have to control your ability to think and remember information. While it may take time, you can begin taking steps today to beat anxiety.

Just as your first hint that you may be struggling with anxiety comes from the physical symptoms, the first step to treating it is also physical. Rest is crucial for having a clear, strong mind. If you are tired, it is much easier to give in to anxiety. But if you establish good sleep habits, your body and mind will be ready to perform optimally, without the strain of exhaustion. Additionally, sleeping well helps you to retain information better, so you're more likely to recall the answers when you see the test questions.

Getting good sleep means more than going to bed on time. It's important to allow your brain time to relax. Take study breaks from time to time so it doesn't get overworked, and don't study right before bed. Take time to rest your mind before trying to rest your body, or you may find it difficult to fall asleep.

> **Review Video: The Importance of Sleep for Your Brain**
> Visit mometrix.com/academy and enter code: 319338

Along with sleep, other aspects of physical health are important in preparing for a test. Good nutrition is vital for good brain function. Sugary foods and drinks may give a burst of energy but this burst is followed by a crash, both physically and emotionally. Instead, fuel your body with protein and vitamin-rich foods.

Also, drink plenty of water. Dehydration can lead to headaches and exhaustion, especially if your brain is already under stress from the rigors of the test. Particularly if your test is a long one, drink water during the breaks. And if possible, take an energy-boosting snack to eat between sections.

> **Review Video: How Diet Can Affect your Mood**
> Visit mometrix.com/academy and enter code: 624317

Along with sleep and diet, a third important part of physical health is exercise. Maintaining a steady workout schedule is helpful, but even taking 5-minute study breaks to walk can help get your blood pumping faster and clear your head. Exercise also releases endorphins, which contribute to a positive feeling and can help combat test anxiety.

When you nurture your physical health, you are also contributing to your mental health. If your body is healthy, your mind is much more likely to be healthy as well. So take time to rest, nourish your body with healthy food and water, and get moving as much as possible. Taking these physical steps will make you stronger and more able to take the mental steps necessary to overcome test anxiety.

Mental Steps for Beating Test Anxiety

Working on the mental side of test anxiety can be more challenging, but as with the physical side, there are clear steps you can take to overcome it. As mentioned earlier, test anxiety often stems from lack of preparation, so the obvious solution is to prepare for the test. Effective studying may be the most important weapon you have for beating test anxiety, but you can and should employ several other mental tools to combat fear.

First, boost your confidence by reminding yourself of past success—tests or projects that you aced. If you're putting as much effort into preparing for this test as you did for those, there's no reason you should expect to fail here. Work hard to prepare; then trust your preparation.

Second, surround yourself with encouraging people. It can be helpful to find a study group, but be sure that the people you're around will encourage a positive attitude. If you spend time with others who are anxious or cynical, this will only contribute to your own anxiety. Look for others who are motivated to study hard from a desire to succeed, not from a fear of failure.

Third, reward yourself. A test is physically and mentally tiring, even without anxiety, and it can be helpful to have something to look forward to. Plan an activity following the test, regardless of the outcome, such as going to a movie or getting ice cream.

When you are taking the test, if you find yourself beginning to feel anxious, remind yourself that you know the material. Visualize successfully completing the test. Then take a few deep, relaxing breaths and return to it. Work through the questions carefully but with confidence, knowing that you are capable of succeeding.

Developing a healthy mental approach to test taking will also aid in other areas of life. Test anxiety affects more than just the actual test—it can be damaging to your mental health and even contribute to depression. It's important to beat test anxiety before it becomes a problem for more than testing.

> **Review Video: Test Anxiety and Depression**
> Visit mometrix.com/academy and enter code: 904704

Study Strategy

Being prepared for the test is necessary to combat anxiety, but what does being prepared look like? You may study for hours on end and still not feel prepared. What you need is a strategy for test prep. The next few pages outline our recommended steps to help you plan out and conquer the challenge of preparation.

STEP 1: SCOPE OUT THE TEST

Learn everything you can about the format (multiple choice, essay, etc.) and what will be on the test. Gather any study materials, course outlines, or sample exams that may be available. Not only will this help you to prepare, but knowing what to expect can help to alleviate test anxiety.

STEP 2: MAP OUT THE MATERIAL

Look through the textbook or study guide and make note of how many chapters or sections it has. Then divide these over the time you have. For example, if a book has 15 chapters and you have five days to study, you need to cover three chapters each day. Even better, if you have the time, leave an extra day at the end for overall review after you have gone through the material in depth.

If time is limited, you may need to prioritize the material. Look through it and make note of which sections you think you already have a good grasp on, and which need review. While you are studying, skim quickly through the familiar sections and take more time on the challenging parts. Write out your plan so you don't get lost as you go. Having a written plan also helps you feel more in control of the study, so anxiety is less likely to arise from feeling overwhelmed at the amount to cover.

STEP 3: GATHER YOUR TOOLS

Decide what study method works best for you. Do you prefer to highlight in the book as you study and then go back over the highlighted portions? Or do you type out notes of the important information? Or is it helpful to make flashcards that you can carry with you? Assemble the pens, index cards, highlighters, post-it notes, and any other materials you may need so you won't be distracted by getting up to find things while you study.

If you're having a hard time retaining the information or organizing your notes, experiment with different methods. For example, try color-coding by subject with colored pens, highlighters, or post-it notes. If you learn better by hearing, try recording yourself reading your notes so you can listen while in the car, working out, or simply sitting at your desk. Ask a friend to quiz you from your flashcards, or try teaching someone the material to solidify it in your mind.

STEP 4: CREATE YOUR ENVIRONMENT

It's important to avoid distractions while you study. This includes both the obvious distractions like visitors and the subtle distractions like an uncomfortable chair (or a too-comfortable couch that makes you want to fall asleep). Set up the best study environment possible: good lighting and a comfortable work area. If background music helps you focus, you may want to turn it on, but otherwise keep the room quiet. If you are using a computer to take notes, be sure you don't have any other windows open, especially applications like social media, games, or anything else that could distract you. Silence your phone and turn off notifications. Be sure to keep water close by so you stay hydrated while you study (but avoid unhealthy drinks and snacks).

Also, take into account the best time of day to study. Are you freshest first thing in the morning? Try to set aside some time then to work through the material. Is your mind clearer in the afternoon or evening? Schedule your study session then. Another method is to study at the same time of day that you will take the test, so that your brain gets used to working on the material at that time and will be ready to focus at test time.

Step 5: Study!

Once you have done all the study preparation, it's time to settle into the actual studying. Sit down, take a few moments to settle your mind so you can focus, and begin to follow your study plan. Don't give in to distractions or let yourself procrastinate. This is your time to prepare so you'll be ready to fearlessly approach the test. Make the most of the time and stay focused.

Of course, you don't want to burn out. If you study too long you may find that you're not retaining the information very well. Take regular study breaks. For example, taking five minutes out of every hour to walk briskly, breathing deeply and swinging your arms, can help your mind stay fresh.

As you get to the end of each chapter or section, it's a good idea to do a quick review. Remind yourself of what you learned and work on any difficult parts. When you feel that you've mastered the material, move on to the next part. At the end of your study session, briefly skim through your notes again.

But while review is helpful, cramming last minute is NOT. If at all possible, work ahead so that you won't need to fit all your study into the last day. Cramming overloads your brain with more information than it can process and retain, and your tired mind may struggle to recall even previously learned information when it is overwhelmed with last-minute study. Also, the urgent nature of cramming and the stress placed on your brain contribute to anxiety. You'll be more likely to go to the test feeling unprepared and having trouble thinking clearly.

So don't cram, and don't stay up late before the test, even just to review your notes at a leisurely pace. Your brain needs rest more than it needs to go over the information again. In fact, plan to finish your studies by noon or early afternoon the day before the test. Give your brain the rest of the day to relax or focus on other things, and get a good night's sleep. Then you will be fresh for the test and better able to recall what you've studied.

Step 6: Take a Practice Test

Many courses offer sample tests, either online or in the study materials. This is an excellent resource to check whether you have mastered the material, as well as to prepare for the test format and environment.

Check the test format ahead of time: the number of questions, the type (multiple choice, free response, etc.), and the time limit. Then create a plan for working through them. For example, if you have 30 minutes to take a 60-question test, your limit is 30 seconds per question. Spend less time on the questions you know well so that you can take more time on the difficult ones.

If you have time to take several practice tests, take the first one open book, with no time limit. Work through the questions at your own pace and make sure you fully understand them. Gradually work up to taking a test under test conditions: sit at a desk with all study materials put away and set a timer. Pace yourself to make sure you finish the test with time to spare and go back to check your answers if you have time.

After each test, check your answers. On the questions you missed, be sure you understand why you missed them. Did you misread the question (tests can use tricky wording)? Did you forget the information? Or was it something you hadn't learned? Go back and study any shaky areas that the practice tests reveal.

Taking these tests not only helps with your grade, but also aids in combating test anxiety. If you're already used to the test conditions, you're less likely to worry about it, and working through tests until you're scoring well gives you a confidence boost. Go through the practice tests until you feel comfortable, and then you can go into the test knowing that you're ready for it.

Test Tips

On test day, you should be confident, knowing that you've prepared well and are ready to answer the questions. But aside from preparation, there are several test day strategies you can employ to maximize your performance.

First, as stated before, get a good night's sleep the night before the test (and for several nights before that, if possible). Go into the test with a fresh, alert mind rather than staying up late to study.

Try not to change too much about your normal routine on the day of the test. It's important to eat a nutritious breakfast, but if you normally don't eat breakfast at all, consider eating just a protein bar. If you're a coffee drinker, go ahead and have your normal coffee. Just make sure you time it so that the caffeine doesn't wear off right in the middle of your test. Avoid sugary beverages, and drink enough water to stay hydrated but not so much that you need a restroom break 10 minutes into the test. If your test isn't first thing in the morning, consider going for a walk or doing a light workout before the test to get your blood flowing.

Allow yourself enough time to get ready, and leave for the test with plenty of time to spare so you won't have the anxiety of scrambling to arrive in time. Another reason to be early is to select a good seat. It's helpful to sit away from doors and windows, which can be distracting. Find a good seat, get out your supplies, and settle your mind before the test begins.

When the test begins, start by going over the instructions carefully, even if you already know what to expect. Make sure you avoid any careless mistakes by following the directions.

Then begin working through the questions, pacing yourself as you've practiced. If you're not sure on an answer, don't spend too much time on it, and don't let it shake your confidence. Either skip it and come back later, or eliminate as many wrong answers as possible and guess among the remaining ones. Don't dwell on these questions as you continue—put them out of your mind and focus on what lies ahead.

Be sure to read all of the answer choices, even if you're sure the first one is the right answer. Sometimes you'll find a better one if you keep reading. But don't second-guess yourself if you do immediately know the answer. Your gut instinct is usually right. Don't let test anxiety rob you of the information you know.

If you have time at the end of the test (and if the test format allows), go back and review your answers. Be cautious about changing any, since your first instinct tends to be correct, but make sure you didn't misread any of the questions or accidentally mark the wrong answer choice. Look over any you skipped and make an educated guess.

At the end, leave the test feeling confident. You've done your best, so don't waste time worrying about your performance or wishing you could change anything. Instead, celebrate the successful

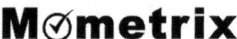

completion of this test. And finally, use this test to learn how to deal with anxiety even better next time.

> **Review Video: 5 Tips to Beat Test Anxiety**
> Visit mometrix.com/academy and enter code: 570656

Important Qualification

Not all anxiety is created equal. If your test anxiety is causing major issues in your life beyond the classroom or testing center, or if you are experiencing troubling physical symptoms related to your anxiety, it may be a sign of a serious physiological or psychological condition. If this sounds like your situation, we strongly encourage you to seek professional help.

Tell Us Your Story

We at Mometrix would like to extend our heartfelt thanks to you for letting us be a part of your journey. It is an honor to serve people from all walks of life, people like you, who are committed to building the best future they can for themselves.

We know that each person's situation is unique. But we also know that, whether you are a young student or a mother of four, you care about working to make your own life and the lives of those around you better.

That's why we want to hear your story.

We want to know why you're taking this test. We want to know about the trials you've gone through to get here. And we want to know about the successes you've experienced after taking and passing your test.

In addition to your story, which can be an inspiration both to us and to others, we value your feedback. We want to know both what you loved about our book and what you think we can improve on.

The team at Mometrix would be absolutely thrilled to hear from you! So please, send us an email at tellusyourstory@mometrix.com or visit us at mometrix.com/tellusyourstory.php and let's stay in touch.

Additional Bonus Material

Due to our efforts to try to keep this book to a manageable length, we've created a link that will give you access to all of your additional bonus material.

> **Please visit**
> **https://www.mometrix.com/bonus948/npadgerprimc** to
> access the information.